Zen Medicine
for Mind and Body

Using Zen Wisdom, Shaolin *Kung Fu* and
Traditional Chinese Medicine

By Shi Xinggui

Better Link Press

This book is edited and designed by the Editorial Committee of *Cultural China* series.

Text by Shi Xinggui
Translation by Zhao Gang
Design by Wang Wei

Copy Editor: Shelly Bryant
Editor: Cao Yue
Editorial Director: Zhang Yicong

Senior Consultants: Sun Yong, Wu Ying, Yang Xinci
Managing Director and Publisher: Wang Youbu

ISBN: 978-1-60220-165-1

Address any comments about *Zen Medicine for Mind and Body: Using Zen Wisdom, Shaolin* Kung Fu *and Traditional Chinese Medicine* to:

Better Link Press
99 Park Ave
New York, NY 10016
USA

or

Shanghai Press and Publishing Development Co., Ltd.
F 7 Donghu Road, Shanghai, China (200031)
Email: comments_betterlinkpress@hotmail.com
Printed in China by Shanghai Donnelley Printing Co., Ltd.

1   3   5   7   9   10   8   6   4   2

The material in this book is provided for informational purposes only and is not intended as medical advice. The information contained in this book should not be used to diagnose or treat any illness, disorder, disease or health problem. Always consult your physician or health care provider before beginning any treatment of any illness, disorder or injury. Use of this book, advice, and information contained in this book is at the sole choice and risk of the reader.

Quanjing provides the images on pages 80, 82, 83, 97, 99, 101, 103, 116, 118, 122, 124, 126, 129, 130 and 137.

Contents

Chapter III
Preventing Physical Disease with Zen Medicine   57

Chapter IV

Curing Physical Illness with Zen Medicine 94

Introduction

Illnesses Come from the Mind, So Treatment Should Too

In his teens, my grandfather became a monk in the Shaolin Temple. There, he practiced martial arts diligently and won the title of Champion of Martial Arts when he later returned to secular life in the late 19th century. However, due to the social upheaval at that time, he returned to his hometown in Dengfeng, Henan Province, only in his old age. Because I was physically weak and often got sick when I was a child, he sent me to the Shaolin Temple to be tutored by Master Dechan.

In the Temple, I learned not only martial arts (*wushu*), which helped me build a strong constitution, but also studied authentic Zen medicine. Originated in the Shaolin Temple, Zen medicine developed under the influence of Zen Buddhism, incorporating meditation, *kung fu*, and medicine. In early times, because the monks often sat for long periods in meditation, their main and collateral channels tended to become blocked, disrupting their blood circulation. Searching for a solution to this problem, they began to practice martial arts and, at the same time, discovered many secret medical formulas based on the rich medicinal materials found on Mount Songshan, where the Temple is located, and developed various folk recipes as the constantly accumulated greater experience in medical treatment. While practicing martial arts, they also created numerous formulas that improved health and had sound medicinal effects. Together, these studies brought about the unique Shaolin Zen medicine, characterized by such medical treatments as *qigong* (breathing exercises), massage, and vital point treatment. Zen medicine, which emphasizes daily health care and cultivation of the body and soul, offers targeted methods for specific medicinal treatment. In addition, the internal exercises for self-cultivation, the external exercises to build the muscles and bones, and the food therapies it created have remained in use until today, bringing many benefits to modern society.

Years later, after graduating from medical school, I became a doctor. I gained some level of fame even as a very young doctor, simply because I utilized Zen medicine in treatment and used the knowledge found in *Bodhidharma Yi Jin Jing* and *Xi Sui Jing* to help patients recover. As the crystallization of medical wisdom lasting for nearly two thousand years, both have extraordinary medical effects. As time went on, I gradually formed my own approach to medicine, combining the wisdom of Buddhism, modern rehabilitation medicine, Zen medicine, and my own experience as a doctor. The extraordinary medical effects thus produced spread far and wide, attracting increasing numbers of patients who sought advice.

I am always eager to excel. An embarrassing event from my childhood demonstrates how eager I was to excel. As part of the training, all the little monks in the Shaolin Temple are made to stand on their heads for as long as the instructor tells them to. A physically weak girl, I often stood longer than most of the boy monks. However, one time, I drank some water before the exercise, and not long after we started I needed a break to visit the washroom. Not wishing to be the first to admit defeat, I tried hard to hold it in. Eventually, urine trickled down my face and mixed with the tears there. This eagerness to excel transformed me into a responsible doctor when I grew up. I worked no less than 16 hours a day in my early years of practice, turning away no patients who came to me for help.

After some time, I began to experience frequent abdominal pain and diarrhea. I never imagined it was cancer. Very soon, I found that I was wrong, and the pain was getting increasingly frequent and the diarrhea increasingly severe. What's worse, I became drastically emaciated. The diagnosis revealed that I had contracted terminal colon cancer, which, by then, had spread to other parts of the body, including the womb, ovary, pelvis, and abdominal wall.

That was 1996, and it changed my fate. Before, I felt that death was something distant, but now it loomed right in front of me. But I really didn't want to die.

Although I grew up in the Shaolin Temple, I did not believe in Buddha or the Bodhisattva. However, lying in my sickbed, I chewed on the word found in Buddhist scriptures, and I suddenly felt that they were true. I silently chanted the name of the Goddess of Mercy again and again, until one day, a miracle happened. In a moment between sleep and waking, I felt the Goddess in white breeze into my room, sprinkling sweet dew-water over me. I grew warm all over, as if I were being electrified. A tingling, supremely comfortable sensation overcame me.

At that moment, I knew I would not die, but must return to the Shaolin Temple.

I was excited by this thought. Childhood memories floated before my eyes. I began to miss the revered Master Dechan and the days when I practiced martial arts, made up prescriptions, and recited words in the scriptures. My desire to live grew even stronger. I came to realize that I needed to practice Buddhism and make up for what I had lost. Later, guided by Monk Suxi, I became a Buddhist monk. Each day after doing exercises, I would devote all my time to reading *The Tripitaka*, a collection of all Buddhist scriptures that includes all the Buddhist disciplines and works of eminent monks from the past and present. I had studied it when I was young, but not systematically. Besides, I had forgotten much of it by this time. Now, I had to act like a newcomer and learn it afresh and systematically.

Reading the scriptures in a calm mood, I was finally

awakened. My obsessive emphasis on gaining personal fame and my eagerness to outdo others in whatever I did had put my mind in turmoil, which eventually resulted in me contracting cancer.

While in the Temple, I was not given a comfortable room to live in, out of consideration for my illness and old age. Instead, I rented a dilapidated hut from a beekeeper. It was close to the Dharma Cave, where the founder of Zen Buddhism faced a wall in meditation for nine full years. From that time on, I started to practice Buddhism in the real sense. Every day, after reading *The Tripitaka*, I went to the Dharma Cave for meditation. Being very fragile, I climbed the mountain path on hands and knees. At first, my gown was soaked with sweat each time I had climbed the first one or two meters. I continued climbing until I was totally exhausted, then I sat, or even lay on the ground, weeping. I did this every day without fail.

I returned to the Temple again after chemotherapy. Having taken medicine every day, I was repulsed by the smell of food. The chemotherapy made it difficult for my intestines to operate properly, and I could only live on gruel. However, the biggest change in me was that I gained some vitality, and I knew I could make it. While maintaining a peaceful state of mind, I persevered in practicing *Bodhidharma Yi Jin Jing*, *Ba Duan Jin* (a 700-year-old *qigong* practice consisting of eight simple movements) and breathing exercises each day. As a result, my health improved with each passing day. Nearly 20 years have passed since I was diagnosed with terminal cancer in 1996, but I am still healthy and full of life.

During this 20 year span, I have combined the ideas of Buddhism and traditional Chinese medicine and have accumulated some experience in treating illnesses and preserving health. I introduced it to my anguished, illness-ridden friends, who found it quite effective. Later, I thought others might benefit from these insights as well. Many people were agitated, unhappy, or even depressed over various small troubles in life, common diseases, or even seemingly for no reason at all.

I am a "talkative" monk. I keep myself busy giving lectures, treating patients, and sharing my experience both inside and outside the Temple. Through my work, many patients have fully recovered and many depressed visitors have been cheered. In hopes of helping more people avoid illness and enable them to have a healthy, happy life, I have put together my reflections on life and my understanding of Buddhist wisdom, effective methods of Zen medicine, and proven recipes, recording them in this book. I sincerely hope that this book will be a gateway to a healthier, happier life.

Shi Xinggui
November 29, 2015

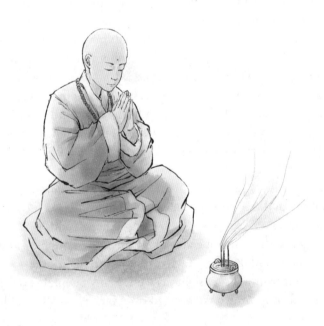

Chapter I
Curing Mental Anxiety to Prevent Physical Disease

In the early years of my medical practice, I was involved in the building of many rehabilitation centers in the US, Germany, and Canada. My pursuit of fame and wealth reached its peak when I was invited to give lectures there. My vanity grew immensely when I saw the large audiences that gathered.

Only after my gradual recovery from cancer did I begin to realize that position and wealth do not belong to us, no matter how much they seem to. When one's life ends, what can he bring with him? We are but passing visitors in this world, and our journey lasts just dozens of years. There is no reason for stubbornness. We must let go. We can only have all these things when the heart is empty enough to hold all.

According to modern scientific research, one's health is determined by many factors, such as heredity, food and drink, emotion, medical care, balance between work and rest, and one's living environment. Among these, heredity makes up 15%, food 10%, emotion 60%, medical care 10%, and others 5%. Obviously, emotion, or state of mind, is key to our health.

This is in line with pulse-taking in traditional Chinese medicine, in which changes in one's emotional state, however small, affect the vital energy and state of the blood, which is displayed in the condition of the pulse. This proves that human emotions and psychology are closely related to disease, as many diseases come from inside. Therefore, one who is mentally ill is physically ill as well. That's why we often hear of someone who falls sick due to anger, anxiety, worry, or annoyance.

One's state of mind affects his health as much as any medical treatment. All diseases are due to one's mental state, and they will be cured once the mental state is properly aligned. According to traditional Chinese medicine, a disease is cured more through general healthcare than through medical treatment, and the key to general healthcare is adjusting the patient's state of mind. In many people's eyes, cancer is incurable. While it is true that many cancer patients die one to two months after a diagnosis is made, there are also many who continue to live a normal life. The moment I was diagnosed with cancer, I thought I should diligently fight it, but I later discovered that I was wrong. Instead of beating my brains out to kill the cancer cells in my body, I assumed a calm, fearless attitude toward the disease. I let it be and kept myself happy and carefree. In this way, my state of mind improved, and so did health.

1. Maintaining Good Spirits

According to traditional Chinese medicine, the essence of life, vital energy, and spirit represent the three aspects of life respectively, i.e. the principle and material basis, the dynamics and energy movement, and the dominator and external symptoms. Being closely linked, even indispensable, to life, they are invaluable to human beings, as they are the prime mover of one's life, the basis for one's health, and the prerequisite for one's career development. Consider whether you have ever seen a successful person looking listless or sighing in despair in public. Of course not! When you are in good spirits, you naturally look sunny and positive, and this mental state will also affect others, such as your business partner, and will pave the way for fruitful conversation. By contrast, a lagging spirit is often associated with negativity, which will attract other negative things, including disease.

How then, can we maintain a good spirit? The most important thing is to present our best state of mind to others.

When I was seriously ill, I was all skin and bones and had little physical strength. However, when there were visitors, I did not hold back when receiving them. Even though I often wept at the afflictions afterwards, I told myself not to impose my own pains and troubles on others.

The second thing one must do to maintain good spirits is to get moving. The human body consists of two kinds of energy, i.e. yin and yang. If we stay inert in the daytime, the yang energy will not be generated. How can we be strong and healthy then? If we keep active at night, the yang energy will not change into the yin energy, and how can we fall asleep that state? Look at the children around you. They scamper around in the day and sleep like a log at night, falling asleep as soon as their heads hit the pillows. Some children don't wake up even if they fall from the bed. This is a perfect example of the balance between yin and yang.

Receiving others with vigor and spirit benefits our body and soul. It also prepares us for a brighter future.

2. Not Enslaved by Material Gain

Mr. Liu, a wealthy lay Buddhist, was diagnosed with liver cancer. He asked me, "I've converted to Buddhism for five or six years now and have chanted Buddhist scriptures each day for about half an hour. How have I contracted cancer? Does Buddha really exist?"

I knew that he was walking the same path I once walked. What he felt was exactly what I felt. I believed that he might have pondered over these questions for some time. When I was in good condition, I devoted myself wholeheartedly to winning personal fame and material comforts everywhere I went, but when I came down with cancer and was confined to bed, I was awakened to the fact that money could not save my life, no matter how much of it I had.

Why are so many people today afflicted by depression,

ZEN MEDICINE FOR MIND AND BODY

anxiety, and delusional disorders? Why do they sleep badly
at night and lose interest in food? The reason is simple. Their
hearts are fatigued and they persist too firmly in their pursuit of
material gain. They feel jealous at others' achievements, wishing
to grab whatever they like for themselves. They are reluctant
to give up smaller benefits, but never fail to chase after and
compete for bigger benefits. They are highly emotional, allowing
no mistakes on the part of their subordinates. Blinded by anger,
they can hardly see their own true nature. According to the
traditional Chinese medicine, anger impairs the liver, causing
diseases.

Most of the people in this world have lost their true nature,
abandoning themselves to the pursuit of fame and material gain.
Some, even after converting to Buddhism for many years, remain
sallow and emaciated, lacking in strength from a young age. This
shows that their worldly nature has remained unchanged. What
they worship and pursue are position, wealth, and fame, which
are precisely the sources of disease. Only when they find their
true selves and live a natural, clean life can they gain physical
health.

3. Being Yourself

Su Shi (1037–1101), an important literary figure in the
Northern Song dynasty (960–1127), once held a post in
Guazhou on the north bank of the Yangtze River, which stood
across from the Jinshan Temple, where his friend, the erudite
Buddhist monk Foyin lived. One day, having achieved some new
understanding of Buddhism through meditation, he composed
the following verse to express what he felt:

I bow in worship to the mightiest of the mighty,
Whose light shines over the whole universe.
Against the winds from eight directions,
I sit undisturbed on the purple lotus.

Joyfully, he asked his servant to send the verse to his friend, expecting some praise from him.

Bold and unrestrained, the verse is indeed well-written. The first two lines indicate that one prostrates himself in worship to the Buddha, the most powerful existence in the universe, whose radiance is felt by all. "Winds from eight directions," in the third line refers to the winds of praise, of ridicule, of slander, of extolment, of material gains, of poverty, of suffering, and of satisfaction, which can disturb the state of mind of Buddhist practitioners. The last two lines, therefore, indicate that one sits on the purple lotus like the Buddha, calm and composed, undisturbed by either praise or ridicule.

After reading the verse, the monk wrote only two words on the same piece of paper, then asked the servant to bring it back. Confident of receiving high praise from the monk, Su Shi hastily read the comment. He flew into a rage when he saw the two words "break wind."

Furious, he took a boat to the other side of the river to reason with his friend, who was waiting for him at the riverside. The moment he saw the monk, Su asked indignantly, "Master, we are good friends. Why did you insult me?"

The monk laughed and answered, "You say you are undisturbed by the eight winds. Why have you been driven to this side of the river by my 'wind'?" Ashamed, Su was speechless.

After some time, Su went to visit the monk again. When they met each other, he asked, "Master, what do I look like?"

"You look like a Buddha," the monk answered. Then the monk asked Su, "What do you think I look like?"

"You look like a pile of shit," replied Su.

Thinking that he had avenged himself, Su was walking on air as he left. Back at home, he lost no time telling this story to his younger sister Su Xiaomei, who after some thought, said that he had lost again this time. Confused, he asked for an explanation. "You're what you think," said his sister. "Since you thought of a pile of shit, you are that shit."

This story indicates that we should not be led by others or affected by what others think of us. We should not feel elated when others praise us, complacent when they flatter us, or irritated when they insult us. We should follow our hearts and not be troubled by external things.

In our daily life, it is not difficult to notice that when we talk about others, we are composed and cheerful, but much less so when we hear others talk about us. This shows that many of us are too mindful of others' opinions and worry that others might laugh at us. We do not know, however, that this can only trouble our minds, which can lead to disease.

But who on earth hasn't done anything laughable, and who on earth is not ridiculous? When have you seen the merciful Buddha laugh at all living things? Then why don't we treat others with mercy and accept them with kindness? Only in this way can we be our true selves, not the self reflected in others' eyes. When our state of mind does not fluctuate with external circumstances, we can rid ourselves of trouble and disease.

4. Prevention Is the Best Cure

I often give lectures in the Temple, sometimes on Buddhism, and other times on disease prevention. The lectures are heartily welcomed. Many of the people who attended my lectures are seriously ill. They arrive on wheelchairs or supported by their families, seeking for comfort. They often asked me directly, "Master, why did I get this disease?"

I usually tell them that the Bodhisattva fears the cause, but not the result, while man fears the result, but not the cause. Knowing that doing evil is the cause of retribution, the Bodhisattva does her best to avoid wrongdoings, however small they might be. By contrast, we consider wrongdoings, especially smaller ones, nothing important, often committing them at will. If we are not fearful of the cause, we must then bear the result when it comes. However, when the result does come, many of us do not choose to bear it, instead complaining and pretending not to know the cause. For instance, to satisfy our appetites, we choose food that is spicy and salty, or meaty and greasy. When we do this, how can we avoid falling ill? It is important, then, to learn to fear the cause. When we find it hard to control our appetites or emotions, we should try to think of its result, which might make us more watchful in the future.

On the other hand, there is no need for us to be so pessimistic when we do fall ill. We should also fear no result, because when we suffer, it means that suffering will soon be over. When we enjoy happiness, it means our happiness is reduced overall. Therefore, we must realize that being ill is a threshold. We are agonized now only because we are trying to cross the threshold. When we do cross it, we are blessed.

5. Keeping Fit through Exercise

Laziness is the source of all disease. When we are in motion, no disease will catch up with us, but when we are lazy, many "diseases of the rich" will find us, such as high blood pressure, hyperlipidemia, and diabetes. *Lü's Commentaries of History*, a Taoist masterpiece from China's Warring States period (475–221 BC) contains such the famous saying, "Being in constant motion, running water is never stale, and a door hinge is never worm-eaten." If a person does not exercise often, his vital energy and blood will not circulate well, and his health will be at risk.

Why are there so many diseases of the rich in modern society? In the final analysis, it is because of the lack of exercise and the comfortable life to common today. We have sofas to rest on at home and cars to drive when we are out, but our muscles don't get enough exercise. Like grass at the foot of the wall that is kept from sunshine, our bodies are soft and weak, lacking reactiveness and a healthy immune system. And disease is sure to take this opportunity to attack. Therefore, people who are reluctant to exercise or who exercise very little are unlikely to enjoy good health. To keep fit and healthy, we need to formulate an exercise plan as early as possible and stick to it every day, making exercising a habit.

6. Avoiding Anger

A woman in her sixties had often listened to my lectures at the Temple, but it had been some time I had seen her. When I did see her again, she was wheelchair bound, pushed to the Temple by her daughter. She did not look well. It turned out that she had just recovered from a serious illness. One day when she was buying vegetables, she had been given a fake 50-*yuan* note. After discovering that it was a fake, she rushed to find the peddler in the vegetable market, but he had left without a trace. Furious, the woman began to feel dizzy. She had a stroke and was hospitalized. What she ultimately lost was not only 50 *yuan*, but more than 10,000 *yuan* in medical charges.

Anger is the source of many diseases. No one likes getting angry, but living in today's complicated society, it is inevitable that we become irritated, resentful, or even hostile because of the unpleasant things we come across.

Anger is not a good thing. Throughout history, many people have died of anger. According to the teaching of traditional Chinese medicine, anger impairs the liver, because it causes liver yang hyperactivity and makes the patient feel dizzy or even spit up blood. Sadly, many patients with heart disease or high blood pressure become angry over trivial things and finally die in an uncontrollable fury.

In fact, to get angry is to get sick. We often say that it is anger that causes illness. If we are so angry, we lose our appetite, we may have stomach troubles. If we feel fidgety or suffer from insomnia, we may develop mental anxiety. If we feel like throwing things, insulting others, or even dying, it may be a sign of liver-related liver depression. If our blood pressure rises and our heartbeat increases, we may develop high blood pressure, heart disease, or cerebrovascular diseases. If a woman gets angry easily, she may develop gynecological diseases such as mastitis and breast lumps.

What's worse, anger also destroys our interpersonal relationship. Once, an older woman came to me saying that her husband had said very ugly things to her. I asked, "Why didn't you answer?"

She said, "If I did, he would have become even angrier. Then both of us would be angry. Why bother doing that? Instead, I come to the Temple to relax."

"You've made the right choice," I said, "because getting angry only makes things more difficult for yourself. If you don't get angry, anger will not find you. If you are angry with your colleagues, you won't be able to do your work. If you get angry with your family, your life will become a mess. The Buddha teaches us several methods of self-adjustment. The first is to step away for a moment, and the second to tell ourselves that if we get angry with others, we are trapped. Finally, we should try to think of what we look like when we get angry. You have instinctively used the first method, so you're quite enlightened."

She was elated when she heard these words, which, though few, had filled her with joy.

7. Controlling Your Emotions

Similarly, people may fall ill because of sorrow or overexcitement. Human beings possess seven emotions, joy, anger, worry, anxiety, grief, fear, and surprise, all of which are closely linked with their internal organs. For example, extreme grief injuries the lungs, extreme fear harms the kidney, and extreme joy taxes the heart. Our health is, therefore, directly determined by our emotional state, and extreme emotions do harm to our physical and psychological health.

The Buddha says, "To follow the path of the Bodhisattva, one must be able to endure humiliations." This indicates that we must remain clam in the face of both setbacks and heavy blows, as well as in success and joy. The Buddha teaches us to control our emotions, neither pleased by external gains nor saddened by personal losses.

Some people become nervous the moment they fall ill, turning in desperation to any doctor they can. In consequence, a minor illness develops into a major one, often as a result of misdiagnosis. Other people, dizzy with their success, immediately become outspoken and reckless, bringing disaster to themselves by hurting others or causing jealousy. Such outcomes grow out of extreme emotion and a chaotic heart. As the most crucial of all organs, if it is in trouble, the heart will fail to control the other internal and external organs, and disaster will naturally ensue.

When I was young, my teacher told me a story. Once there was a farmer whose field was beside an expanse of reeds. Since wild beasts often frequented the reeds, he always patrolled the border area between his field and the reeds with his bow and arrows, to prevent the beasts from destroying his crops.

One day, the farmer went to protect his field again, but the whole day, nothing happened. Towards evening, he was tired. Seeing that nothing would happen, he sat down at the edge of his field for a rest.

Suddenly, he noticed reed catkins flying up into the air from among the reeds. He couldn't help wondering, "I didn't shake the reeds and there's no wind now, so what has made the catkins fly up? There must be some beasts moving among the reed."

Alarmed by this thought, the farmer stood up and looked carefully into the reeds. Only after a long while did he find a tiger scampering around excitedly. Oblivious to the danger nearby, it jumped out of the reeds, exposing itself to the farmer's sight.

"Why is the tiger so excited?" thought the farmer, "it must have captured its prey." Hiding himself, the farmer aimed at where the tiger stood. He shot the arrow as soon as the tiger jumped out again. With a shrilling scream, it fell back among the reeds.

When he went over to see what had happened, the farmer found a tiger with an arrow in its chest and a dead river deer beneath it.

This is exactly the sort of disaster brought on when one gets carried away by extreme joy. Of course, just as extreme joy is not a good thing, neither are extreme grief, anger, anxiety, and fear. Extreme grief can impair the lungs. A Chinese idiom which refers to a state in which ones is "choked with sobs." This serves as a good example. Why does a sobbing person easily become choked? Because his grief leads to depression, which in turn may block his smooth breathing.

In a similar way, extreme anxiety, impairs the spleen. For example, when you anxiously wait for your partner to return home, you are not in the mood to eat. Even if you do eat several mouthfuls, the food seems bland. What's worse, anxiety results in a gloomy mood, which, if it carries on too long, will cause nervous disorders and a decrease in the secretion of digestive juice. This, in turn, will lead to other symptoms, such as a loss of appetite, panting, weariness, fatigue, and depression. In addition, overanxiety is another reason for poor blood circulation, slowness of thought, or even thoughts of suicide.

Extreme fear injures the kidney. When frightened, one's legs may shake or he may urinate frequently. Some may even wet their pants. All these conditions have to do with kidney function.

In order to maintain our health, we must maintain a peaceful state of mind. My secret lies in just two words: keep smiling. Whatever we encounter, we must face it with a smile. There is no need to take things too seriously, whether good or bad. What we need is to take a deep breath, adjust our mood, and be calm. If we are open-minded, tolerant, composed, and benevolent in our handling of worldly matters, we will get fewer diseases and more blessings.

8. Not Focusing on Your Illness

Being ill need not be terrifying. What's terrifying is one's attitude toward the illness.

Once, I came across a patient suffering from heart disease and mental anxiety. A little over 60, she said to me the moment she saw me, "Master, with this heart disease, I could leave the world any time."

I led her to the southwest corner of the Temple, where there was a pile of sand that had been left after a building was completed.

I asked her to take a handful of the sand. Somewhat confused, she did as I said. I instructed her to hold on tightly so that the sand would not flow out.

However, the more tightly she tried to close her fist, the more the sand escaped through her fingers.

"You see the sand?" I said, hoping to inspire her. "It is your illness. The tighter you hold it, or the more you want to control it, the faster it escapes you. Similarly, the more attention you pay to your illness, the more serious it will become."

Suddenly enlightened, the woman thanked me profusely and left.

Unexpectedly, she came to me again three months later to update me on her story. She said that when she heard what I said the previous time, she felt a bang of enlightenment, but mental anxieties are rarely healed all at once. Sometimes, she just could not help but think about her illness. Then, one day, she went to that pile of sand again, collected some of it in a paper bag, kowtowed to the Buddha, and went back home.

At home, she put the sand into several smaller paper bags and brought one wherever she went. Every time she thought of her illness and felt pessimistic about life, she would hold the sand in her hand, watching it flow through her fingers, pondering my words.

Later, she did not need the sand anymore. When she was faced with unpleasant things in life, including her illness, my words would come to her unprompted, and she would immediately tell herself not to be bothered by excessive worry. As a result, she felt happy from then on. Some time later, she told others about her story during morning exercises, and many elderly people benefitted from her experience.

Therefore, falling need not be scary at all. As long as we adopt a correct attitude toward it, we can enjoy our work and life unimpeded.

9. What You Do for Others Will Eventually Benefit Yourself

A farmer opened a store on a city street. Before long, he found that business was bad at this location, and the street was pot-holed and dotted with broken bricks and stones. Puzzled, he consulted the neighboring shopkeeper, who told him that poor road conditions would slow down the pedestrians and vehicles, which would in turn increase business opportunities, since more people would enter the stores. Disapproving of this logic, the farmer removed the bricks and stones on the roads and had the surface leveled. As a result, the once deserted street now became busy and prosperous, and business opportunities increased dramatically. When asked how this had happened, the farmer explained, "When the road is poor, people will bypass it. With fewer people coming, how can business opportunities increase?"

It is always wise to treat others well, which will lead to oneself being treated well. Concern for others is the biggest investment in one's own interests.

Another story demonstrates the opposite side of this principle. An old carpenter was retiring soon. Feeling reluctant to part with him, his boss asked him to build one more house before he left. Though he agreed, the carpenter was not happy, thinking that he did not need to obey his boss anymore. He was careless with his work, using poor materials and muddling through his work. To his surprise, when the house was finally built, the boss told him that it was a retirement gift for him. The carpenter was ashamed and regretful. He did not realize that he had been building his own house, but it was too late.

In fact, all the good things you do for others will eventually benefit yourself. For example, if you are asked to do more work, don't complain, because it is a chance for you to temper yourself, and in time, you'll be entrusted with important tasks. While you might seem to have suffered loss in doing good deeds and helping others, you will be blessed in the end. Therefore, whatever you do for others, do your best, because you are doing it for yourself. Only in this way can you accumulate your own reward in heaven.

10. Living a Slower Life

Two monks, one old and the other young, were each carrying two buckets of water on a shoulder pole from the foot of a hill to their temple on the hilltop. Thinking that he could have more time for rest if he arrived at the destination earlier, the young monk quickened his steps and reached the temple in half an hour. The old monk, instead, remained unhurried, climbing the hill more gradually and reaching the top in an hour. "Master, why didn't you ramp up your efforts like I did and arrive earlier so you could get rest?" the young monk asked.

"You were indeed faster," answered his master, "but you're just cooling down now, aren't you? In this sense, aren't we arriving at the hilltop at the same time?"

Similar examples can be seen in many areas of our life. Many people are always in a hurry on their way to work. Sometimes, they even cross the street when the light is red. But when they reach their workplaces, they sit panting heavily, and it takes them a long time to cool down. The same happens when they

go home after work. While they may get home several minutes
earlier, they but are often too exhausted to spend time with
their families. So what difference is there whether they get home
earlier and later? This being the case, why not walk slower?

Most of us have a similar approach to life. In our early years,
we earn money at the cost of our health, and in the second half,
we use that money to buy health. As a result, we are kept on the
run all our lives. If you think about it, this sort of life is no more
desirable than a long simple life. When they fall ill, many people
eagerly look forward to an immediate recovery, but this is rarely
possible, because haste makes waste.

I once came across a boy with recurrent fever. When I
asked about its cause, his mother said, "Previously, he ran a
fever of 39 ℃. He was hospitalized in the morning, but his fever
had not dropped by evening. Worried and anxious, his father
yelled at the nurse for not doing her work properly. At this, the
doctor immediately wrote a prescription and asked the nurse
to bring down the fever with the medicine prescribed. After
more than one hour of intravenous drip, his fever abated. With
two more days of infusion, his temperature was normal and he
was discharged from hospital. But once he got home, the fever
recurred, lingering for days."

I knew the reason immediately. "How could you let his
father yell at the nurse?" I said to the mother. "Fever is a self-
protecting mechanism of the body. It shows that the immune
system in the body is fighting the germs. Instead of doing harm
to the child's body, a controlled fever benefits it greatly. With
antibiotics, it is easy to bring down the fever, but antibiotics are
a double-edged sword, killing both good and bad cells in the
body, and consequently, the patient becomes physically weaker.
Your son could have overcome the fever without taking medicine,
but because of your anxiety and yelling, the doctor had to
use antibiotics instead. That's why he is now plagued with this
recurrent fever."

We should slow down the pace of our life. When we are angry or impatient, or if our relatives are falling ill, we should tell ourselves, "I am now at the crossroads and the light is red. If I don't slow down, I'm sure to encounter more serious trouble."

11. Happiness in Contentment

The most fundamental human desires are wealth, sex, fame, food, and sleep. As mortal beings, we naturally have desires, and some of them are not bad at all. For example, the lack of desire for food will cause anorexia, and the lack of desire for sleep will lead to insomnia. If he is utterly pessimistic, a patient is unlikely to be healed. Therefore, an appropriate amount of desire is good, but too much desire will cause trouble, agony, and restlessness.

Mr. Wang originally ran several restaurants, but when he came to me, he had nothing left to his name. Wang was a common child from a common urban workers' family, and his mother even lost her job. But he was smart even as a child, and very insightful. At 25, he married a woman who owned a small restaurant. With this foundation, he worked hard for ten years and became the owner of five large restaurants.

Last year, one of his good friends told him that by investing in a project, he could have his wealth doubled within a year. Impressed, he mortgaged all his restaurants and put the money into the project. Unfortunately, the investment failed and he lost several million *yuan*. He was so depressed he attempted suicide. His wife, who often came to the Temple to offer incense, asked me to give her husband some guidance.

"Let me tell you a story," I said to Mr. Wang. "Long, long ago, there was an old fisherman, who lived with his wife in a shabby hut on the seaside. Every day, he cast the net into the sea to catch fish while his wife wove yarn. But his luck was bad, and he did not catch any fish for several months. One day, he finally caught a small goldfish. Unexpectedly, the fish begged him to set it free and promised to grant him whatever wish he might imagine. The old fisherman said that he wanted nothing, and he freed the fish into the sea."

"Master," interrupted Mr. Wang, "I heard this story."

I smiled. This was normal, since many people knew this story. But I asked him to finish it.

Mr. Wang continued, "Back at home, when the old fisherman told this to his wife, she started cursing and forced him to ask the fish for a new wooden basin, and it was granted. Then she asked for a wooden house and a noblewoman's title, which also came true. Finally, the insatiable woman even wanted to be queen, waited on by the goldfish. Running out of patience, the fish ordered everything to return to what it had been. In the end, the old woman still lived on the seaside with her broken wooden basin in her shabby wooden hut."

"Are you the old woman in the story?" I asked him when he finished the story. He seemed to be inspired by the story.

"I know everything about you." I continued, "You were smart as a child. You saw through many worldly things, but not into your own heart. You couldn't control your heart and, like a balloon, it grew bigger and bigger, until it finally burst. This is like climbing a mountain. Though you're good enough to conquer the mountain, when you finally stand at its top, you don't know to stop and appreciate the infinite views below, the sunrise the next morning, and the flowers and grass that cover the mountain. Instead, you walk ahead one more step, but unfortunately, that means you're beginning to go down the mountain."

Intelligent people know how to control their desire. After their normal desire is met, they are no longer affected by greed. When you are well-fed and well-clothed, you might as well consider how many beautiful things in this world have you missed while you kept yourself busy every day. Why not put down the things you are doing, calm down, and enjoy the beauty of this moment?

12. Cherishing What You Have

Many people, some of whom are successful in most people's eyes, complain to me that they are not happy and that life is meaningless. Some young people even consider suicide.

Once, a man in his thirties came to me, saying that he was under great pressure and was unhappy. He said he came from the countryside and lived in the city after graduating from the university. I asked whether he had more money now than in his childhood. He answered that when he was young, his family was very poor. Then I pursued, "Do you think you had a happy childhood?"

He thought for a while and answered, "We were poor at that time, but when I recall those days, there are still many happy memories, such as catching fish in the river and climbing trees to catch cicadas."

"You're right," I said. "When do people feel happy? It is today, this moment. However, many people do not know how to live their present lives well. When they are young, they think their childhood was happier, and when they are middle aged, they think they were happier in their youth. When they are old and riddled with disease, they think their middle-aged life was happier. Never wait until tomorrow to recall the happiness of today."

"Master, this is very convincing," the man said, relieved.

Many people believe that "the poor have their worries, and so do the rich." However, I often tell them that "the poor have their happiness, and so do the rich." Happiness knows no class or border. It is deeply rooted in each of us, but we simply lack the eyes to see it.

According to a Buddhist scripture, there was once a wealthy person who was depressed every day and did not know what happiness was. One day, he decided to set out and look for happiness, carrying a bag of golden coins on his back. He said he would give the bag of coins to anyone who could tell him how to find happiness, but he could not find anything to make him happy.

Later, he was told to seek an eminent monk in a temple at the top of a mountain. He went to the temple and poured out his troubles to the monk, but the monk continued in his meditation and gave the man no regard. The man talked and talked until he finally fell asleep. When he awoke, he found both the monk and his bag of coins were gone. Greatly saddened, the man wept, thinking it was unfortunate to have lost the bag of golden coins before he had found happiness. Unwilling to give it up, he searched everywhere for the monk. Totally exhausted, he finally returned to temple, only to find that the monk and his bag were still there. Immediately, he was beside himself with joy.

Only then did the monk opened his eyes. "You already have happiness in yourself," said he. "Why do you take such pains to find it?"

The reason many people do not experience happiness is that they do not know how to cherish what they already have. Aren't our partners, friends, and children the source of our happiness? But too often, we choose to turn a blind eye to them, giving up the happiness we already have, and in this way, we are abandoned to groundless moaning and groaning. The Buddha says that what is lost is lost. Therefore, only when we learn to cherish what we already have now can we understand the meaning of life and the needs of the human nature, and then our lives can be filled with happiness and sunshine.

Chapter II
Curing Mental Anxiety through Zen Medicine

The biggest reason for my success in fighting against cancer is that I experienced true happiness. In those days, though tortured by the disease, I was extremely happy when I cultivated myself, basking in the brightness and warmth of the sun. Each night, when the moon shed its soothing light on my hut, I felt very happy as well, because the Goddess of the Moon was pacifying my mind. Every time I felt I could no longer continue, I was encouraged by Bodhidharma, who had once meditated in that cave for nine years. When I was recovering, I tilled the land to grow crops, cooked, exercised, and meditated, and the disease left my body.

I know another cancer patient who was cured spontaneously. He had a job, but he stopped working after falling ill. Refusing to stay idle, he came up with an idea to keep himself busy—he swept the grounds of the whole residential area every day. At first, his family did not want him to do this, but after reconsidering, they decided to leave him to himself. Unexpectedly, this work led the old man to become increasingly vigorous, and his cancer was finally cured.

Therefore, just as smiling is recognized universally, happiness is the panacea to all diseases. It's true everybody is busy today, but when you have free moments, you might as well recall those happy times in your life. This simple activity will cure many underlying health problems that trouble you, including insomnia, anxiety, depression, and even some more serious diseases.

1. Managing Your Life with Industry and Frugality

Many people ask why, after living a frugal life, they can't accumulate any wealth. In fact, being frugal and being industrious are both complementary and indispensable. We are bound to be poor if we practice frugality alone, and we will have nothing to our names if we focus solely on industry.

Let me begin with a story.

In the old days, people preferred to hang a tablet above their gates, on which were written two words in parallel, industry and frugality. Once when an old man was on his deathbed, he hoped his sons would remember the virtue of industry and frugality, and so divided the tablet in two, giving industry to his older son and frugality to his younger son.

Later, it turned out that the older son worked diligently, but knew no frugality, while the younger son was frugal, but not hardworking. Consequently, both became poor. Finally, the brothers decided to put the two words together, and in that way, becoming both industrious and thrifty, they grew wealthy.

In real life, there are many who uphold only one of the two words. Such people generally do not live well. Some become wealthy doing business, but instead of buying things good for use, they buy anything that is expensive. Eventually, they use up their money and return to poverty. To them, their past riches and honor are nothing more than a fond dream.

Others are exactly the opposite. Although they are frugal, they are simply too lazy, living solely on the money left by their parents. Being frugal alone does not help, and in time, the entire fortune is depleted.

A Buddhist proverb says, "Industry and kindness generate wealth and happiness, while laziness and evil result in poverty and bitterness." Being industrious and frugal is an indispensable virtue. Before we practice this principle, we need to understand it thoroughly.

2. A Calm Mood Brings Good Luck

To conduct ourselves in society, we should be aware of ways to cultivate our hearts and temperament. Nothing we do will fail if done calmly. If a general in the front can remain composed at crucial moments, he then make clear-headed decisions. If a businessman can have a peaceful mind in dealing with matters of vital interest, he is certain to be on the winning side. If a student can stay cool during his examinations, he will score high marks. Therefore, maintaining calm mood at critical moments is particularly commendable. It is also the secret of preserving health. According to traditional Chinese medicine, anger impairs the liver, which will in turn impair the heart. Therefore, we should try to remain calm and undisturbed in dealing with all things, because getting angry means we are punishing ourselves with the mistakes of others.

To clearly judge a person's moral standards, scholarship, and competence is very difficult, but a calm mood is an essential quality we should cultivate.

Let me illustrate with a story. Zeng Guofan (1811–1872) and Li Hongzhang (1823–1901) were among the four greatest ministers in the late Qing dynasty (1644–1911). Once, the latter recommended Liu Mingchuan (1836–1896) and two other scholars to the Zeng, who invited them to his residence for an interview. Instead of showing up at the appointed time, he kept them waiting in the living room and observed them in secret. The two scholars grew impatient and kept complaining, but Liu remained composed, appreciating the calligraphic works and paintings hanging on the wall. It goes without saying that Liu was the one who was recruited.

To conclude, the ability to keep composed is essential to our success. Getting angry easily will eventually impair our health, without which everything else is but a dream. Moreover, if we conduct ourselves in a calm, undisturbed manner, others will consider us trustworthy and steadfast, and the road ahead will become smoother. Otherwise, we will alienate ourselves from others and become unapproachable.

3. Breaking Away from Constraints

Some elderly people tell me that they are not free at home, or that they often quarrel with their daughters-in-law. Some younger people say that the companies they work for limit their personal development. In fact, the root of all these troubles is the heart. Only when the heart is free can the body be free.

When the Bodhidharma arrived in the eastern land, he saw a cage hanging from the beam of a house, inside which was a beautiful bird. The bird chirped continually as soon as it caught sight of the Bodhidharma, who understood that it was asking him how it could get out of the cage. He said, "You must lie down with your legs stretched out and your eyes closed."

After a while, when the owner of the bird came in, the bird did what the Bodhidharma said, stretching its legs out, closing its eyes, and pretending to be dead. Surprised at the sudden death of his favorite bird, the owner immediately opened the cage to see what had happened to it. Seizing the opportunity, the bird flew out and gained its freedom.

There are people who feel frustrated at work. They keep complaining like the bird in the cage. But the Buddha teaches us to change our fate by actively changing the environment we are in. Therefore, if we change our state of mind and work hard, we can earn a good reputation in our work environment. In time, some better companies will come for us and we can then break away from the confinements of our former environment.

4. Forgiving Others

Once when he was taking a walk at night in the temple courtyard, an old monk saw a chair at the edge of the wall. He immediately knew that a monk had climbed over the wall, which was against the rules of the temple. The old monk moved the chair away and squatted against the wall. After a short while, a young monk climbed onto the wall. Stepping on the back of the old monk, he jumped into the courtyard.

Instead of scolding him in a sharp voice, the old monk quietly told him to go and put on more clothes, since it was the middle of the night and getting chilly. He chose to forgive his disciple, because he knew that forgiveness is a form of silent education. From then on, the young monk kept the temple rules. His master forgave him just one mistake, but what the master got in turn was his respect for himself and for the Buddha.

I heard another story. In an American market, a Chinese woman ran a very good business, causing jealousy from other sellers. Consciously or unconsciously, they all swept their trash to the front of the woman's stall. Instead of complaining, the woman swept it to the corner of her stall, smiling.

After watching her for several days, a Mexican woman selling vegetables there, could not help asking her, "Why didn't you get angry at them when they swept their trash right in front of your stall?"

Smiling, the woman answered, "In my country, during the Spring Festival, people will sweep the trash into their houses. The more trash they have, the more money they will make in the next year. How can I refuse it now that everyone here is sending money my way? Don't you see that my business is becoming better and better?" From then on, the woman saw no trash in front of her stall.

This Chinese woman wisely forgave others, creating a harmonious environment for herself. Since harmony brings wealth, her business improved greatly. What would have happened if she had retaliated? The answer is obvious.

When you make a mistake, you expect forgiveness and support from others. Likewise, when others make a mistake, they expect the same from you. Open your window of forgiveness. You will find that when you forgive, you become forgivable yourself, and the number of your friends will quickly increase.

5. Learning to Be Grateful

When he was a child in the Tang dynasty (618–907), Master Longtan was very poor, making a living by selling bread and having no place to live. Seeing this, Master Daowu lent him a small hut beside his temple. To express his gratitude, the boy sent ten pieces of bread to Master Daowu each day. Master Daowu often gave one back, then blessed Master Longtan.

Perplexed, he asked the Master one day why he gave back one piece of bread each time. "Since the bread is given by you," said the Master, "is there anything wrong with me giving it back to you?"

Suddenly enlightened, the boy decided to be converted, and he eventually became an eminent monk himself.

We should learn to use what we take from others to benefit others, and what we take from society to benefit society. A blessing is the greatest when it benefits both sides. This is also a truth of life.

At the most critical moment of my illness, I was at my last gasp, weighing only 39 kilograms, and the number of the white blood cells in a milliliter of my blood fell below 1,800. When I went back to the Foguang Temple, many nuns prayed for me, offering me spiritual support. As a Buddhist and doctor, I took great pleasure in giving them lectures, because I knew my second life was given by them and I should do what I could to repay their kindness.

Being grateful is one of the most beautiful things in this world. In Buddhism, there is a term "transference," which means giving your most cherished thing to others. In fact, all the achievements, such as a bowl of food or a cup of water, are the result of combined efforts. However successful you might be, you must remain grateful, as your wealth is not created by you alone, but by all your employees as well.

6. Thinking from Others' Perspective

It is only natural that there may be misunderstandings, conflicts, and quarrels between people, because we all tend to think ourselves correct and others wrong. However, different people may have different perspectives, even when viewing the same thing. From their perspective, they are certainly correct. If we all argue for our own points of view, conflicts are bound to occur. In fact, many controversies are due to different perspectives, which can be successfully resolved if we can think from others' perspective.

The Buddha says that other people are our best mirrors. We will be treated the way we treat others. If we do not think for others, others will not think for us either. Therefore, if we learn to think from others' perspective, we will have a totally new life.

In whatever we do, we should learn to put ourselves in another's shoes. Only in this way can we find their real needs and understand and help them. This will also relieve our own troubles and pains and bring less trouble to others. With more understanding and less annoyance, we are sure to live a happier, healthier life.

7. Unburdening Your Mind

Every one of us is under pressure. The poor have pressure just making a living, and the rich rack their brains to become richer. Often, we may think of our own pressures alone, but ignore those of others. In fact, it is impossible for anyone to live without pressure.

Why do some people live a happy, wealthy life while others live a miserable, poor life? The key lies in discarding our mental burdens. Though life is full of burdens, if we learn to let them go, our lives will be different. When we are burdened, it is difficult to move forward, but if we put our burdens down, we are sure to go farther.

Another story will illustrate the point. On his way to do business down the mountain, a Buddhist master saw an old woman sobbing in a corner. He went over and asked, "Why are you weeping so sadly?"

"Master, you don't know," answered the woman. "I have two daughters, one married to an umbrella seller and the other a shoe seller. In fine days, I worry about my first daughter, since she may not sell her umbrellas, and on rainy days, I worry about my second daughter, because no one will then buy her shoes. I can't help feeling sad at the thought of this."

"Oh, I see," said the master. "You might as well think, when it rains, one of your daughters' umbrellas will sell well, and your other daughter's shoes will do well when the weather is fine. If you think this way, every day, whether it is sunny or rainy, will be a happy day." Convinced by these words, the woman wept no more, but felt happy every day.

The old woman in the story was unhappy because of her heavy mental burden, but when she put it down, she became happy and carefree.

Life's journey is long and arduous. Do you prefer to discard your burdens and enjoy the view on the way, or trudge along with a heavy bundle on your back? Even if what is in the bundle can prevent you from hunger and cold, don't you think you have lived your life in vain if you simply move on with your head lowered and miss the view? If this is the case, why not unburden your mind and start fresh? In fact, you will find that everything will be smooth and successful without these mental burdens.

Zhuangzi (c. 369–286 BC), an ancient Chinese Taoist saint, knew this well. Untroubled by worldly fame and gains, the fate of the country, or setbacks in life, he achieved absolute freedom at heart, just like the fluttering butterfly and the soaring roc.

Try to imagine, if he had failed to unburden his mind, how could he have attained such a realm beyond the grasp of others, taken his wife's death philosophically, and befriended people based on morality and justice? The ancients are gone, never to return, but their philosophical idea of freeing oneself from mental burdens has become deep-rooted and will be passed down across generations.

Overall, life is long and the burden we carry will accumulate as time passes. If we do not learn to unburden ourselves, we will eventually collapse under its weight, and so will our body, career, and family. Only when we move forward without mental burdens can we have a better life.

8. Giving Help without Expecting Returns

As things keep changing in our lives, we must rely on help from friends and families. Those who give us sincere help are important people in our lives. Here, I emphasize the word "sincere," because only sincere help counts. Giving help in exchange for personal gain does not add to one's merit and virtue at all.

Nothing in our lives can help us accumulate merit except offering selfless help to others. The Buddha says that if you help two people in your life, your cultivation will be refined, and if you help a dozen, you will be immensely blessed.

A sincere helper will do his utmost to help others, expecting neither returns nor gains. When you give help without asking for returns, you increase your own blessings. Only in this way will you have others' sincere help when you are in trouble.

An ant fell into a river while drinking from it. He tried his best to swim to the bank, but to no avail. Spinning in place, he struggled in despair. A large bird hunting for food nearby saw him. Sympathetic to the ant's plight, he picked up a little branch with his beak and cast it to the ant. Climbing on the branch, the ant finally got safely to the bank.

When the ant was drying himself on the grass near the river, he heard some footsteps. He saw a hunter with a gun silently approaching the bird. Quickly, the ant climbed onto the hunter's toes, then into his pants. The ant bit the hunter hard just before he fired. The hunter screamed, and his bullet missed his target. Alarmed by the gunfire, the bird fluttered its wings and flew away. In this story, the ant and the bird saved each other's life.

When the bird helped the ant, he did it sincerely, expecting no return. Eventually, the ant helped him escape disaster.

To conclude, don't do things based on your own benefit alone. Learn to love others and sincerely help them. By doing so you can win others' hearts.

9. Disregarding Personal Gains or Losses

I was extremely happy when I recovered from cancer, because I had learned not to care about my own gains and losses. Bad things will always happen in our lives, and when we suffer losses, we cannot help but feel sad. We question why the world is so unfair and why bad things happen to us. However, there are no answers for these questions. If we continue to look at things this way, we will inevitably fall into depression.

We might well ask ourselves what's so good about having things. Everything in this world will be eventually gone. What's bad about not having things? Life itself is illusory. Between having and not having, we can find life. Sorrow and pleasure are determined by the state of mind we have based on our gains or losses. We cannot enjoy happiness unless we take gains and losses lightly. Since losses are inevitable, those who take them too seriously will lose even more. By contrast, those who care little for that which is lost will ultimately gain more.

In China's Warring States period, there was an old man named Sai Weng, who had many horses. One day, one of his horses was missing, and his neighbors came to his home to comfort him. Smiling, he said perhaps it was a good thing. The neighbors thought that he was just trying to comfort himself. Several days later, his horse returned, bringing with it another fine horse. The neighbors then offered their congratulations. However, the old man remained undisturbed, saying that this turn of events might not be necessarily a good thing. Later, the old man's son fell from the horse and broke his leg. When others consoled him, the old man said, "Although my son broke his leg, this might be a blessing to him, since he might have saved his life instead." Those around him all thought otherwise, but before long, when the enemies invaded the border, all the young men except for the old man's son were enlisted into the army, and most of them died on the battlefield. The son's broken leg had spared him from military service.

This story demonstrates that disasters and blessings are interchangeable. When a good thing happens, we should not feel too happy, because extreme joy begets sorrow. When a bad thing happens, we might as well accept it calmly and not be too concerned about it, because bliss often arises out of the depth of misfortune.

We must know that life is never perfect. As we grow older, we may become discontent, flighty, or impetuous due to pressure from work and society. We tend to sigh over the hardships and difficulty of life, complaining that we have given too much in exchange for too little. However, constant complaints will erode both body and soul, driving happiness and health even farther away. It is only when we have a peaceful state of mind and care little about gains and losses can we live a pleasant, peaceful life.

10. Being Ready to Cooperate with Others

There is no lack of "lone wolves" in this world, those who attend to everything personally and communicate with and listen to no one else. When in trouble, they often feel they have no alternative but endure it all by themselves, but in fact, it is totally unnecessary for them to do so. They can avoid many detours if they will cooperate with others, listen to other's advice, and bravely accept other's help. In today's competitive society, even if they are talented, their individual strength is limited. The key to success is often the ability to combine the wisdom of many.

In the final analysis, Buddhist cultivation is the cultivation of the heart, because each heart is an independent entity. Like a magnet, the heart can help us amass fame and wealth. Therefore, if we know how to draw on collective wisdom through communication and cooperation, then many magnets can come together to form a powerful magnetic field. Even though others may not be as smart or learned as we are, they can offer some suggestions, because they may look at an issue from different perspectives from our own and see what we may not be able to see. Based on our combined wisdom, discussion, and analysis, we are sure to formulate the best plan.

To sum up, drawing on collective wisdom is humans' most extraordinary ability and the engine for social progress. It can bring about miracles and open new possibilities, and it can stimulate our greatest potential. Our future hinges upon united wisdom.

11. Harboring Fewer Worldly Desires

A young man who wishes to learn the secret of being indifferent to fame and fortune once traveled a great distance to visit a castle in which an old wise man lived. After listening to the young man, the old man asked him to move about the castle carrying a spoon filled with oil and not spill a drop of it.

When he returned, the old man found that not a single drop of oil had been spilt. But when he asked the young man what he had seen on the way, the young man said, "I focused solely on the spoon and saw nothing else." Then, the old man asked him to move around the castle again, but this time to be aware of everything in the castle.

When he came back again, the young man described the things in the castle in great detail, but every last drop of the oil in the spoon was gone. Then the old man said, "Worldly affairs are as complex as the grass and trees in the castle, and one's body and soul are like the oil in the spoon. Some people live far away in mountains seeking after a simple, tranquil life, not knowing that living in seclusion does not necessarily lead to purity of mind. Faced with temptations, they may be easily attracted to the world again. When you moved around the castle the first time, the oil did not spill because you concentrated totally on the oil, but the second time, you were distracted, and all the oil was spilt. Though it is foolish to indulge in fame and wealth, withdrawal from society is not necessarily right either. Only if you can remain firm and steadfast after experiencing all the ups and downs in the world can you live a tranquil and undisturbed life and hold firm your spoon of oil."

This story is highly philosophical. The spoon of oil is insignificant, but it is something under our control, such as health, family, friends, or career. Whatever we do, we should avoid being taken captive by our blind, crazy material desires, while on the other hand, we should not go to such extremes as to shun the world, or we will lose ourselves and miss the most beautiful views in life.

Having less desire is an attitude toward life. It is not passive waiting or allowing ourselves to be manipulated by fate. It is, instead, seeking balance in life. Only with this attitude can we fully enjoy the life's grandeur.

12. Keeping a Low Profile

A lion was having a rest under a large tree when he saw an ant walking quickly. Out of curiosity, he asked, "Little fellow, where are you going?"

"To the grassland on that side of the mountain," answered the ant. "It's so beautiful there."

Interested, the lion said, "Climb on my back and lead the way. Let's go there together." Seeing that the ant hesitated, the lion continued, "I run much faster than you."

"Mr. Lion," said the ant, "it's not that I don't like your company, but that you can't possibly reach the grassland."

Enraged, the lion said, "Are there any places in this world I can't reach? It's that side of the mountain, isn't it? Take your time, then. I'll go there myself."

Very soon, the lion came to a bottomless cliff several dozen meters wide. Across the cliff was the beautiful grassland. After hesitating for a long time, the lion finally decided he could not risk jumping over the cliff. But he did not wish to bypass the cliff from the nearby valley, either. In the end, he went back, dejected.

Several days later, the ant also reached the cliff. He climbed to the bottom of the valley and then up the cliff along the slope, reaching the grassland he had longed for.

The ant was small and weak, but he kept a low profile, bypassing the cliff and venturing through the valley, finally reaching the grassland successfully. The lion was the king of animals, and he was powerful, but he refused to lower himself, so could only sigh at the beautiful grassland from a distance.

Many people today are like this. They feel conceited receiving higher education or enjoying success at work. They are not willing to eat at the same table with their nannies, or to mix with their subordinates, or to do manual work, since they consider that these things are beneath them. But with this attitude, they are unlikely to increase their chances for success.

The sea becomes boundless when it receives water from many rivers, but this is only because it is in a lower position than the river. If you wish to climb the peak of success at work, you must learn to keep a low profile. No matter how numerous or outstanding your achievements, you should still mix with others as an equal. You should be able to see their merits and admit your own shortcomings, which will allow you to accumulate more positive energy for yourself.

While floating in the air, a grain of sand is but a bit of dust. But when it is on the ground, it is part of the soil. Dust and soil are from the same source, but the heights they occupy give them different values. There is a Chinese saying, "One loses by pride and gains by modesty." If you put yourself in a high position, you will inevitably feel lonely there, but if you allow yourself to occupy a lower position, you can incorporate everything that is useful to make yourself stronger.

13. Being Thankful for Criticism

No one is perfect, including me. Impatience and anxiety over gains and losses once almost deprived me of my life. Later, it was several revered monks who pointed this out to me directly. They said to me, "You are already ill, but you're still thinking of fame and wealth. This will certainly make your illness worse. It's high time you slowed down and nursed yourself back to health."

In my sick bed, I considered their words for a long time, then I decided to rid myself of all distractions and concentrate on my illness. I'm still alive today, thanks to their sincere criticism and instruction. Most people might have only said nice things to me, not pointing out my shortcomings for fear of offending me.

According to the *Daodejing*, an ancient Chinese philosophical work, faithful words are not nice and nice words are not faithful. In most cases, people love to hear nice words. For example, you are happy when others say you're smart or beautiful, but you usually can't bear to hear others criticize you.

Being criticized is not a bad thing. You should thank others for pointing out your shortcomings, because this can help you improve. Therefore, when you are criticized, accept the criticism calmly and don't harbor any grudge or hatred, because only through others' criticisms can you truly understand yourself.

It is also important to remember that others will criticize

you only when they think you are worthy of the criticism. If they don't care about you, they won't take the risk to criticize you at all.

In the Warring States period, Mozi (dates unknown), a revered ancient Chinese saint, once reprimanded his disciple Geng Zhuzi. Feeling himself wronged, the disciple complained, "Why do you always reprove me so severely when I'm the one who makes the fewest mistakes?"

"If you are climbing a hill in a carriage drawn by a horse and a goat," asked Mozi, "will you whip the horse or the goat to gain speed?"

"Of course, the horse," replied his disciple.

"Why don't you whip the goat?" Mozi pursued.

"There's no use whipping the goat, because the horse is stronger and faster," answered the disciple.

Then Mozi said seriously, "I'm strict with you, because you, like the horse, are worthy of my criticism."

Praise might be false, so you can generally ignore it. Criticisms are mostly genuine, so you must be thankful to those who criticize you. Just as bitter medicine cures sickness, unpalatable advice benefits your conduct. Being able to receive criticism humbly is a virtue, because as Chinese ancient sages said, "I am happy when others criticize me. I will correct my mistakes, if there are any, and keep a record if none has been committed." It is important to be thankful to those who criticize you, whether the criticism is reasonable or not, because that is what will drive you forward.

14. Accepting the Reality and Changing Yourself

Upon learning that I had cancer, I was depressed for nearly a month. My mind was cluttered, thinking that I would soon leave this world. I didn't know whether anyone would remember me after my death. In other words, I simply couldn't accept reality. As this state of mind continued, I found myself becoming so weak I did not have the strength to speak. I realized that this condition had to be changed. After much thought, I began to cheer up. Why couldn't I live a more relaxing life in my remaining days? Having accepted this reality, I gradually began to feel better. This experience demonstrated how big an influence emotion has on health.

The following story resembles my own experience. Though it is lengthy, it is worth repeating.

A man roving alone in a forest was suddenly met with a starving tiger. When the tiger roared and pounced upon him, the man ran with all his might and speed. In hot pursuit, the tiger finally cornered him at the edge of a cliff. "I would rather jump down the cliff than be bit to death by the tiger. There might be a ray of hope if I jump down," thought the man.

Without hesitation, he hurled himself down the cliff. Fortunately, he was stuck on a plum tree growing on the cliff. Before he could even congratulate himself on his luck, he heard a huge roar from the bottom of the cliff. Looking down, he found a fierce lion looking up at him. His heart trembled as it roared. But on second thought, he accepted the facts. "There's no need to fear. The lion and tiger are both fierce beasts. Is there any difference in being eaten by either of them?"

Just as he regained his calm, he heard another sound and found that a pair of mice, one white and the other black, were biting with great force at the plum tree. He was panicked, but soon felt at ease again. "Just let it be. When the tree is bit off, I will fall and die, but this is much better than being eaten by the lion."

Totally relaxed, he felt a bit hungry. Seeing that the plums on the tree were good and ripe, he picked some and ate them, feeling that they were the best plums he had ever had in his life. When he was full, he decided to have a good sleep before he died, so he soon fell sound asleep on a thick triangle-shaped branch.

When he awoke, he found that the mice were gone, and so were the tiger and lion. Carefully, he climbed up to the top of the cliff and escaped from danger. What he didn't know was that when he was sound asleep, the hungry tiger became impatient and jumped down the cliff with a huge roar, scaring away the mice. At the bottom of the cliff, the tiger fought violently with the lion, and after both were injured, they left.

We will inevitably encounter setbacks in our lives, such as diseases, difficulties at work, and family troubles. Like the hungry tiger and the fierce lion in the story, they will either pursue us or wait for us up ahead. When this happens, all we can do is let nature take its course. When we learn to accept things as they are, we may be greeted with a pleasant surprise.

In other words, when things cannot be changed, we may as well accept them and adapt to them. This is wisdom, which can make our lives shine with brilliance. To live a splendid life, we should muster up our courage when we need to persevere, and accept the reality when we need to do that.

The Buddha says that only when we face reality can we transcend it. In fact, sometimes, we might gain more than we had originally hoped for if we gladly accept what cannot be changed, rather than stubbornly haggling over it. Those who are unable to accept reality will never have peace of mind, but will be entangled in endless trouble.

We must know that the world will not change to suit us, and the only way out is to accept reality and change ourselves.

15. Playing up Strengths and Avoiding Weaknesses

Ever since I converted to Buddhism, many people have come to me with their difficulties, especially difficulties at work. After each lecture, many people circle round me, asking me to give them advice. After careful and long-time observation, I have discovered that many of them are not competent for their roles at work, due largely to their "shortcomings." When they see others perform well, they consider themselves "too foolish." When this state of mind continues, they gradually fall even further behind.

In fact, it is not that they are too foolish, but that they are not fit for the particular kind of work they are doing. In another position, they might have left others far behind. A tortoise cannot compete with a hare on land, but it is much faster in water.

I have seen a painting, entitled *Don't Try to Teach the Donkey to Sing*. In the painting, there is a pianist who plays while enthusiastically teaching a donkey to sing. The implied meaning is profound. Hardworking as it is, the donkey is not fit for singing, so there's no use teaching it to sing. Like the donkey, we all have our strengths and weaknesses, and we must learn to play up our strengths and avoid our weaknesses if we are to realize our life's value.

Ms. Liu graduated from a business school in a well-known university, then got a job in a private company doing public relations. However, since she was oversensitive and reluctant to communicate with others, she gained no recognition from her colleagues even after several years of work. This caused her much sorrow.

When she told me her problems, I said, "Ms. Liu, since you are so sensitive to details, why don't you get a certificate and work as an accountant or auditor?" She followed my advice and later became an accountant. When we communicated recently, she told me that she is doing very well at her new job.

As everything has two sides, so our weakness may be the reverse side of our strengths. As long as we can place ourselves in a position where we can play up our strengths, we will feel like a fish in water.

The Buddha says, "Don't wait until you are praised to believe in yourself." We must not wait to believe in our strengths, for we only live once. It is important to find a job we are fit for as soon as possible and find fulfillment in that position.

16. Being a Good Listener

When we speak, we wish others to be good listeners, but when others speak, we are often inattentive. This problem might prevent us from progressing smoothly.

If we are careful enough, it is not difficult to find that either the eminent monks in real life or the Buddhas and Bodhisattvas on TV speak very little when they converse with others. Are they not good with words? Of course that cannot be the case. They are so erudite and eloquent and when they do speak that even stubborn stones nod in agreement. They speak less because they have lent their ears to others, and this is exactly why they have achieved so much.

I once heard a story from a fellow Buddhist. An envoy from a small country presented three identical gold figurines to the Chinese emperor as tribute, but he also raised a question for the emperor, asking which of the three was most valuable. The emperor used all means possible to find a solution, having them examined by experienced jewelers, weighing them, and comparing the workmanship, but they were exactly the same. What should the emperor do now? How was it possible that no one in this entire country could answer such a simple question?

Finally, an old minister came up with a solution. He inserted a piece of straw into each of the three figurines. The first straw came in one ear of the first figurine, then out the other ear. The second straw went through the mouth of the second figurine, then fell out of it. The third straw passed through the throat of the third figurine and fell into its stomach soundlessly. The minister concluded that the third figurine was the most valuable of all.

This answer was correct. In fact, the third gold figurine in this story is comparable to those who are good listeners. They listen attentively, digest the information they get, then sum up the experience for their own use.

Only when we are good listeners can we know ourselves and others well and make fewer mistakes based on judicious judgment. Listening to others will also remove misunderstandings, make us work more efficiently, and offer us a more harmonious working environment.

In summary, the most powerful person is not necessarily the most eloquent, but he is surely the best listener. The Buddha gives us two ears and one mouth, which shows that he wants us to listen more and speak less. When we are good at listening to others, we are a step closer to success.

17. Being Modest

A wandering mouse made his home at the top of a Buddhist tower. He found that life in the tower was very happy, since he could have fun running across each floor and could enjoy the abundant sacrifices offered. He was also able to enjoy some privileges no one else could imagine, such as chewing on the unknown Buddhist scriptures and leaving his excrement on the head of the sacred Buddha whenever he wanted. Seeing the believers devotedly kowtow to the Buddha enshrouded in intoxicating incense smoke, he would sniff his nose and laugh secretly. "You silly human beings! Why kowtow to a dead statue?"

One day, a hungry wild cat broke into the tower and caught the mouse. Before the cat ate it, the mouse protested, "You can't eat me. You should kowtow to me, because I represent the Buddha!"

"People kowtowed to you because of the position you occupied, not because of who you were," answered the cat. With that, he swallowed the mouse in one gulp.

You might have heard this story, but have you ever thought carefully about how it applies to you? You might have been doing what the mouse did. Many people feel complacent when others show respect to them, thinking that they are the elites seated on some pedestal. They don't know that people respect them because they wish to get something out of them. Have these people ever considered how others will treat them if they were ousted from positions of power?

The family of Zeng Guofan has lasted for over 190 years, producing more than 240 famous descendants and not a single good-for-nothing. Why is this? Because it is the tradition of the family to adhere to six words: industry, piety, thrift, benevolence, perseverance, and modesty. Children of the family have been required not to put on any bureaucratic airs, not to sit on a sedan chair, not to ask others to serve them food and tea, not to mistreat the servants, not to slight the neighbors, and not to throw their weight around. That is why the Zeng family has remained prosperous for generations.

We should never be complacent. At work, when others respectfully ask for our help, we should treat them with respect, too. Then when we are in need, they will not make things difficult for us. If we wield our power and prestige, our road ahead will become increasingly narrow.

18. Having a Clear Conscience

Buddhism advocates doing good deeds. However, it is often difficult to distinguish between good and evil. For instance, suppose Country A is hit by a natural disaster and its people live a miserable life due to a scarcity of natural resources. To help them out of this situation, the king leads his army to invade Country B, which has to rise to defend itself. Superficially, both countries are killing, and they kill for the benefit of their peoples. But which is good and which is evil?

On the surface, it is difficult to give an answer. However, when judging, we should not only look at the surface of a problem, but how an idea is conceived, which is essential when learning Buddhism. The natural disaster suffered by Country A cannot become the cause for its invasion of Country B.

Invading another country in the name of bringing good to its
own people is equivalent to robbing others to feed oneself. Both
are illegitimate. Therefore, in this case, Country A is evil, and
Country B is good.

In fact, if we look at an issue from different perspectives
or standpoints, we will understand good and evil differently.
Therefore, we should not base our judgment of good and
evil only on superficial factors. The key lies in how an idea is
conceived. If it is conceived out of mercy, kindness, and honesty,
it is a good deed. Therefore, before we do anything, we need to
ask whether we do it out of a clear conscience. If the answer is
yes, we may feel free to do it, and it will eventually benefit us.

19. Ridding Yourself of Bad Habits

A seedling cannot grow into a large, straight tree unless it is
carefully trimmed. A piece of wood cannot become useful unless
it is polished by the carpenter. Likewise, a person can amount
to nothing without cultivating himself. Self-cultivation means
correcting all the deviations in our thought, conception, body,
language, and behavior. It also means ridding ourselves of bad
habits and wrong ideas.

We know all the rules of being healthy, but we still cannot
maintain our health. The reason is that we have not followed
these rules strictly and rid ourselves of our bad habits. For
example, we all know that smoking causes lung cancer, but we
still smoke. We all know that eating less is good to our health,
yet we still eat and drink gluttonously. Although we are clear
about the result of these things, we count on luck and act as we
please. Being ignorant and fearless is not something to be feared,
what is truly frightening is being informed and still fearless of
the consequences of our actions.

Like Buddhist cultivation, health preservation cannot
succeed if we do not possess great wisdom and willpower. How
can we rid ourselves of bad habits? We can write a list of our

bad habits or behaviors on a piece of paper and check each item against that is characteristic of ourselves. We then must consider why we have these habits. When we are clear about the causes, we will find that they bring us only harm and nothing good. Then we will naturally have the motivation to correct these bad habits.

Nevertheless, we should not be overhasty in correcting bad habits when they are many and stubborn, as haste makes waste. Instead, we should correct them bit by bit and one at a time. This way, we will gradually improve our personalities and consciously follow good habits.

20. Persevering in Medical Treatment

A friend of mine, a gentleman in his sixties, had been learning Buddhism for many years. His health remained poor after his retirement. He did not get sick so often, but he was always in low spirits. According to him, he aged faster than others. I taught him to pound his back with his own fists, regardless of when or where he was.

According to traditional Chinese medicine, the back is where the Governing Vessel and bladder meridian (see page 142) are located, and it is also the place all human internal organs hinge on. Therefore, pounding the back regularly can invigorate the yang energy, dredge the channel, promote blood circulation, and harmonize the internal organs. It also relieves fatigue, calms the heart, and tranquilizes the mind. Only when the yang energy is sufficient, the blood is in good circulation, and the internal organs are in harmony can we become full of spirit and energy.

As good as this method was, my friend told me after he had tried it for three months that the effect was not obvious. When I asked more, I learned that he did not persevere with the treatment, doing it only when he thought of it. This, of course, did not work, because "diseases come on horseback, but go away on foot through continued treatment." Although methods of supplementing the yang energy abound in traditional Chinese medicine, none will be effective unless the patient perseveres in the treatment.

According to a philosopher, two species in the world can finally reach the top of the pyramid. One is the eagle, and the other is the snail. The former is highly talented and can soar into the sky easily. The latter, though mediocre in talent, can also succeed in reaching the summit. What he depends on is nothing but perseverance.

The most difficult thing in the world is to persevere. This is also true in medical treatment. Seeing no obvious effect after two or three days of treatment by a doctor, many patients wish to change doctors or medicine, not knowing that they must persevere with a particular recipe before it takes effect. In fact, most of the time, it is not that the medicine is not effective, but that we lack perseverance in treatment.

21. Time Management

Samantabhadra Bodhisattva once said, "As each day passes, our lifespan is reduced by a day. What can we speak of happily when we are waiting for death like the fish in a drying river? We should be urgent in our cultivation, as if the fire were burning on our heads. Faced with the uncertainty of life, we must not be slack in our cultivation."

When I laid on my sickbed, this line of scripture appeared in my mind again and again. For several days, I repeated it. Gradually, I came to realize why some people were healthy and successful, while I was confined to bed by illness. This was because they had allocated their time more appropriately than I did. Those who are healthy use their time on self-cultivation, while those who are sick use it on an unhealthy lifestyle.

Having figured this out, I understood that my priority had to be cultivation of the mind, so, I began to spend more time exercising and chanting Buddhist scriptures. As I improved, I also sought to benefit others. Apart from self-cultivation, I also spent time treating patients and giving lectures. As a result, my health has continued to improve.

In my lectures, I often ask, "Is it possible for us to succeed at work, take good care of our families, and maintain good health at the same time?" The answer is, "Yes, it is possible. As long as we allocate our time appropriately, we can make ourselves better and more successful."

22. Venting Negative Emotion Where It Is Due

Most of the time, life is not satisfactory. It is best if we can take it easy and maintain a good state of mind. However, when bad things happen to us, most of us cannot face it calmly and will feel angry, downcast, and even scared. Holding onto depressed emotions does harm to our health.

So what should we do? We need to give vent to these negative emotions. Why? Because our psychology and physiology are often interrelated and interactive. Psychological disorders will affect physiological health.

For example, if a person has experienced a high pressure environment or depression for a prolonged period, the changes in his hormone secretion and muscle tone will prevent his immune system from staying in its best working condition. This will in turn reduce his resistance against diseases. This is also why people in a bad mood are prone to infectious diseases and people subject to long-term stress are cancer-prone.

However, we must choose the right means to vent our emotions, such as hiking with friends, swimming, or shouting in a secluded place. When we articulate what we wish to say, we will feel relaxed and the pressure of life, along with the effects of negative things from the past, will naturally leave us. Another good way is to pour out our grievances to someone whom we trust and who understands us. After that, we will feel that the world is instantly gets refreshed.

In addition, we can also ease our pressure through exercise, such as jogging, playing ball games, or with a punching bag. All these will help us let out negative emotions. The thing we choose to punch can be a pillow or a rubber doll. When we do punch, punch hard, but remember not to hurt yourself.

All in all, the purpose of such exercise is to give vent to the depressed emotions and resume psychological balance and health. When we are psychologically healthy, we naturally feel comfortable, which will in turn benefit our physical health.

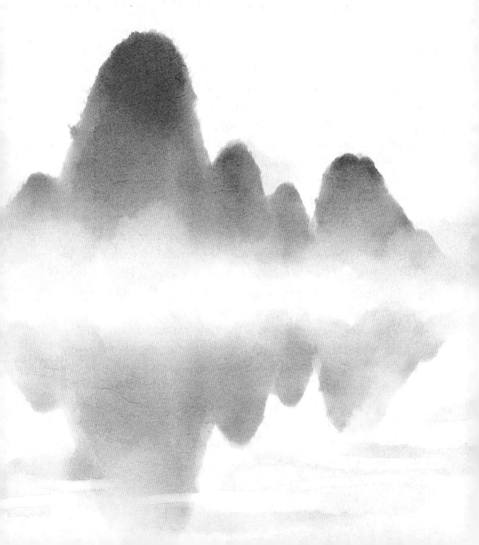

Chapter III
Preventing Physical Disease with Zen Medicine

1. Shaolin Internal Exercises

At the mention of the Shaolin Temple, many people will think of Shaolin *kung fu*, a kind of martial arts developed by Shaolin monks across generations to combat nature, aging, and disease.

In many people's eyes, Shaolin *kung fu* is quite mysterious, but it is actually nothing more than a set of exercises developed on the basis of human physiological and psychological characteristics aimed at disease prevention and health preserving.

Shaolin *kung fu* starts with the internal exercises, which are laid out here.

Preparational Movements

Choose a clean, quiet, spacious place with fresh air, and begin at sunrise. Stand facing the sun, with your feet shoulder-width apart, your arms hanging naturally by your sides, and your eyes facing straightly ahead. Keep your body relaxed, but not sagging. Maintain this position for about three minutes.

Now try to imagine that your head connects the sky and your feet are deeply rooted in the ground. The energy of the earth then reaches the elixir field through the Yongquan point (see next page), and the energy of the sun goes down to the same region through the Baihui point.

Gathering Natural Energy

Movements: Raise your arms on both sides, palms down, until they are level with the shoulders. Turn the wrists, palms facing

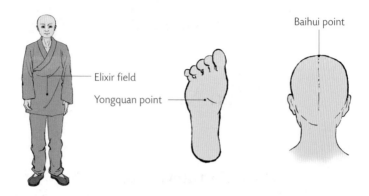

each other, then move the palms inside towards the chest, as if holding a large ball. Turn the palms down when they are about 20 centimeters away from the chest, and then simultaneously push both palms downward, directing the energy to the elixir field. Repeat this set of movements at least 10 times.

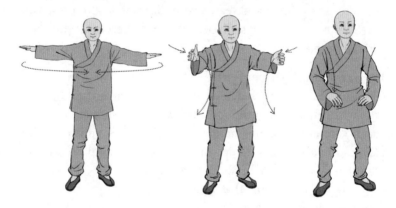

Breathing: Inhalation starts when the arms are raised and finishes when they move inside towards the chest. Exhalation occurs as the palms are turned and pushed downwards. While moving the arms towards the chest, try to imagine that the energy of nature goes into your body through the Laogong point and pores, then gathers at the Danzhong point. While exhaling, direct the energy in your chest toward the elixir field.

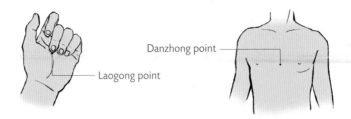

Danzhong point

Laogong point

Gathering the Sun's Energy

Movements: Raise the arms from both sides of the hip, palms up, as if holding a big ball, and then move them towards the top of the head. When the fingertips are nearly touching each other, the palms will naturally face down. Complete the movements by pushing the hands down from the top of the head to the chest, then to the elixir field. Repeat this set of movements at least 10 times.

Breathing: Inhale while raising the hands from both sides of the body, and exhale while they are being pushed down. Try to imagine that the energy of the sun, like a white tiger dashing down a mountain, enters the Baihui point, then is directed from there into the elixir field as the hands are pushed down.

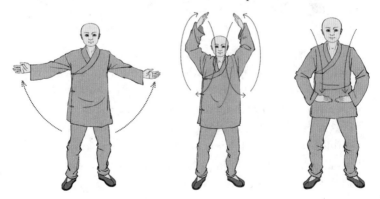

Gathering the Earth's Energy

Movements: Raise the hands from both sides of the body, palms facing the front. When the hands are level with the shoulders, withdraw them towards the elixir field as if holding a big ball.

Meanwhile, bend down, bunch up the body, and flex the neck.
Lift the left knee up against the chest with the foot high up, like a
crane walking. Bend the right knee to stabilize the body. After the
left foot touches the ground firmly, straighten the back and get
up. Complete the movements by following the same steps with
the right leg. Repeat this set of movements at least 10 times.

Breathing: Inhale while raising the arms, and exhale while
moving the arms inside toward the chest. Guide the energy of
the earth to the elixir field through the Yongquan point.

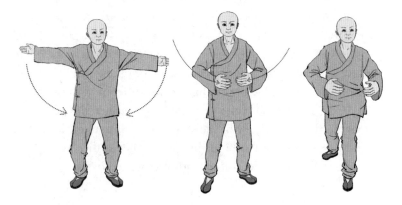

After these three sets of movements are completed, stand
resting for one to two minutes, then rub your hands, wipe your
face, and pat your body all over, so that the pores will close to
prevent any external pathogens from invading the body.

This is the foundation of the Shaolin internal exercises.
Doing this every day will keep you full of vigor, strong, and
healthy, allowing you to enjoy a longer life. As the most
fundamental exercises, they are well suited to beginners.

2. The Six-Word Breathing Technique

Sakyamuni, founder of Buddhism, once asked his disciples, "Do
you know the meaning of life?"

One disciple answered, "Life is the period of time that starts from birth and ends at death."

The Buddha shook his head.

Another disciple answered, "Life lies in food. It ends when there is no food."

The Buddha shook his head again.

Perplexed, they asked, "Then what's your elevated opinion, master?"

"Life," answered the Buddha with a smile, "is between breaths."

What did Sakyamuni mean? Life is unpredictable. Who knows what will happen in the next second? We should cherish the present time and not waste a minute or even a second. Those who are healthy should make full use of their time, working hard and making progress. Those who are ill should summon their courage to defeat their diseases.

A six-word breathing technique, which has benefitted many disciples, is practiced in the Shaolin Temple. It is used both as a method of exercise and of illness treatment. Its technique is laid out here.

Using the *Xu* Breathing Technique to Exhale

This technique nurses the liver and treats liver diseases.

Movements: First, sit cross-legged, clench your fists lightly, and rest them on the knees. Then, take a deep breath and "whistle" it out while leaning back and circling your body

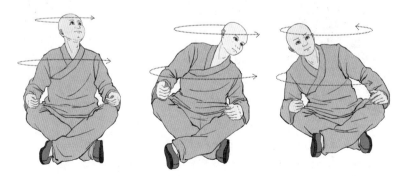

once from left to right. Finish the circle when the exhalation is completed. Finally, take another breath and circle your body from right to left in the same way. Repeat the set of movements six times each morning and evening.

Using the *He* Breathing Technique to Inhale

He is the sound you utter when you smile out of happiness. According to traditional Chinese medicine, the heart corresponds to joy through emotion. For this reason, using the *he* breathing technique to exhale can benefit the heart.

Movements: Sit cross-legged in a natural pose, with your thumbs on the Jiquan points, crossing your hands on your chest so that you hit the right Jiquan point with your left thumb and the left Jiquan point with your right thumb. Take a deep breath and use the *he* breathing technique to exhale, pressing your thumbs against the Jiquan points with force. Loosen your thumbs when the exhalation is finished. Repeat this set of movements six times. After the exhaling, rub the antithenar eminence with your thumb until it warms up.

The Jiquan point is easy to find. It is located at the center of the armpit, where an artery pulses vigorously.

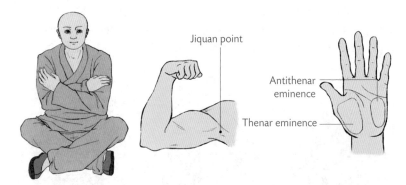

Jiquan point

Antithenar eminence

Thenar eminence

The *he* breathing technique can also be used to enhance the heart function of those who suffer from heart disease, such as tightness in the chest, shortness of breath, palpitations, and angina.

Movements: Assume a sitting posture, placing your right hand on the precordium, with the center of your right palm on the left nipple and the middle finger on the Jiquan point, then place your left hand on top of your right hand. Turn your body from left to right while using the *he* breathing technique to exhale. At the same time, push down heavily with both hands, and press the projection area of the mitral valve (located between the 3rd and 4th ribs) hard with the thenar eminence of your right hand, simultaneously pressing the Jiquan point with

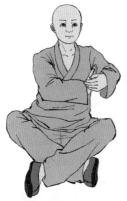

your middle finger. After the exhalation is complete, turn your body to the right and straighten your back, pushing up the tip of your heart (located at the intersection of the 5th rib and the vertical line starting from the middle point of the left clavicle), with the antithenar eminence of your right hand while inhaling.

Repeat this set of movements for as many times as you like.

Using the *Hu* Breathing Technique to Exhale

This technique benefits the spleen and stomach.

Movements: Sit cross-legged in a natural position, clasping your hands over your stomach, and inhale. Raise your hands to the chest and push them outward in front of you, using the *hu* breathing technique to exhale simultaneously. Complete the exhalation when your hands have reached their maximum extension. Turn your palms down and inhale. Repeat this set of movement six times daily.

Then, press down hard from the Shangwan point to the Xiawan point with overlapping hands (placing left hand inside right hand for male, and right hand inside left hand for female) six times. Maintain your hand posture and pull left while you push right on the stomach area. As you pull left, place your hands around the Zhangmen point below the left rib, and pull (push for males) hard with the four fingers of the right hand (left hand for males) from below the left rib to the Zhangmen point on the right side of your body. When pushing right, push (pull for males) hard with the base of your right palm (left fingers for males) from the right Zhangmen point to the left Zhangmen point until an intestinal sound is heard. Use the *hu* breathing technique to exhale when pulling or pushing and inhale when you change between the right and left ribs.

Lastly, massage the Zhongwan point first anti-clockwise and then clockwise 36 times each with overlapping palms.

The Shangwan and Xiawan points are easy to find. Feeling upward from the abdomen, you will find two bones, the lowest ribs. Continue to move upward and you will discover that the two ribs meet at a point, which is called the xiphoid. The distance between the xiphoid and the navel is 8 body inches and right in the middle of that distance (4 body inches from the navel) is the Zhongwan point. One body inch above the Zhongwan point is the Shangwan point, and two body inches above the navel is the Xiawan point. (In this book, we use "body inches" to locate points. The width between the right and left sides of the middle thumb joint is one body inch.)

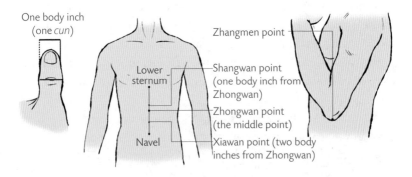

One body inch
(one *cun*)

Lower
sternum

Navel

Zhangmen point

Shangwan point
(one body inch from
Zhongwan)

Zhongwan point
(the middle point)

Xiawan point (two body
inches from Zhongwan)

The Zhangmen point can be found by employing a rather interesting method. Raise a hand and place the center of the palm on the face. The Zhangmen point is exactly at the tip of the elbow.

Using the *Si* Breathing Technique to Exhale

This technique helps clear away the heat in your lungs.

Movements: Sit cross-legged in a natural position and cross your hands over your chest, with your right hand on your left shoulder and your left hand on your right shoulder, and with your right middle finger on the left Jianjing point and your left middle finger on the right Jianjing point. Take a deep breath first, and then use the *si* breathing technique to exhale. While exhaling, turn your waist to the left, completing the exhalation when your waist reaches the point farthest left. Press the Jianjing point hard when you exhale. Repeat the method, turning your waist to the right. After doing this set of movements several times, you will feel the tip of your nose and your upper lips start to get warm. In this method, alongside the breathing techniques, you should rub the Jianjing point, which can dispel wind and clear heat. Used together, they are particularly effective in clearing lung heat.

The Jianjing point is easy to find. Feel from your nipple upward to the top of your shoulder and press it with a finger,

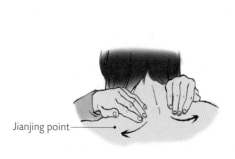

Jianjing point

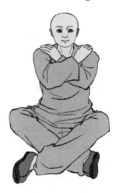

you will find a small depression, which hurts a little when pressed. This is where the Jianjing point is located.

When you catch a cold or have a dry nose and sore throat, you can practice this exercise until you begin to sweat slightly. It is effective for preventing colds.

Using the *Chui* Breathing Technique to Exhale

In traditional Chinese medicine, our five internal organs, the heart, liver, spleen, lung, and kidney, correspond to the five emotions. Of them, the kidney stores will, or aspiration and willpower. It also stores essence and generates intelligence. The kidney, then, relates closely to human intelligence and willpower. This technique can raise your energy levels.

When we reach middle age, the function of our kidneys begins to decline, as do our memories. In addition, since the kidney governs will, our willpower also begins to decrease along with the decline of our kidney function. There are people who get bored sitting before their writing desks even a short time, once they are older. This is in fact a matter of their willpower. If we can nourish our kidneys well, our willpower will increase, and so will our memories.

In the six-word breathing technique, the *chui* breathing technique is unparalleled in nourishing the kidney. The method is simple. Sit on the bed with straightened legs. Take a deep breath and bend forward, catching your feet with your hands. Put your thumbs on the Taichong points and the other fingers on the pelma, with the middle fingers on the Yongquan points. Press hard on the points, extend your feet forward, and point your toes upward inline with your legs. Now hold your breath until it reaches your waist. When you feel warmth in the waist, your kidney is nourished. When you can hold your breath no more, use the *chui* breathing technique to exhale as you straighten your back. Repeat this set of movement at least six times.

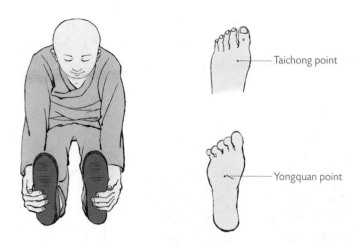

Taichong point

Yongquan point

If you have difficulty bending down, you can lie on your back in the bed and put your hands on both sides of the body in a natural pose. Then, move your toes backwards and your heels forwards, take a deep breath and hold it until it reaches your waist. Use the *chui* breathing technique to exhale when you can hold the breath no more, exhaling as long as your body permits. Repeat this set of movement at least six times.

Using the *Xi* Breathing Technique to Exhale

There is an invisible organ in our body called *sanjiao*, or triple energizers. The upper energizer governs the heart and lung, the middle energizer, the spleen, stomach, liver, and gallbladder, and the lower energizer, the kidney, intestines, small intestines, and urinary bladder. The three energizers are the water channels of these organs. Like expressways, they link all the internal organs, making the transportation from top to bottom smooth. This technique can improve your constitution.

Today, many people are in a state of suboptimal health, tortured by decreased memory, various pains, and dizziness. They would be advised to try the *xi* breathing technique.

Movements: Assume a sitting posture and place the hands in front of the abdomen, palms upward and fingertips facing each other, as if holding something. While inhaling, move the palms slowly upward to the chest, keeping level with the Danzhong point. Then, use the *xi* breathing technique to exhale, turn the palms, and move them close to the thighs. Repeat this set of movement at least six times.

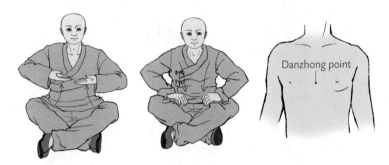

After I got colon cancer, I persevered in practicing the *xi* breathing technique, and it helped me recover.

3. Taking a Walk in a Forest

The concept of vital energy or *qi* is frequently encountered in traditional Chinese medicine. But what is this vital energy? It is a mixture of information, material, and energy, and it exists in all things on earth. The word "aura" is in fact an aspect of the vital energy in traditional Chinese medicine. A tree has its aura, which is its innate property.

For example, the property of the pine is tenacity and uprightness. Therefore, exercising in a pine forest can help strengthen tendons and bones. If you often feel sore in waist and legs or suffer from arthritis, you should try exercising in a pine forest, which will help you obtain the vital energy of pines and increase the effectiveness of your exercise.

The pine can also be used as medicine. Pine needles can invigorate blood circulation, relieve gout, rheumatic pains, and traumatic injuries, and also promote joint health. If you suffer from gout, you can collect some pine needles, boil them in water, and soak your feet in the water, which is very effective treatment for gout. If you contract periarthritis of shoulder and cervical spondylosis, you can boil the pine needles and drink the water in place of tea.

A cypress forest has other unique functions. If you have trouble with your lung, such as a cough, chronic bronchitis, bronchial asthma, and shortness of breath, you can exercise in a cypress forest. Alternatively, a pillow filled with cypress seeds can help improve insomnia. You can collect some cypress seeds in a cypress forest, dry them for one or two days, and put them into your pillow. Using this pillow for several days will cure your insomnia.

Cypress seeds cures insomnia, because the platycladi seed in it is a type of traditional Chinese medicine. According to doctors of traditional Chinese medicine, the platycladi seed benefits the heart, kidney, and large intestine meridians and can calm the heart, tranquilize the mind, stimulate bowel movements, and help in the elimination of waste. According to *Compendium of Materia Medica*, an ancient Chinese medical classic, the platycladi seed "can help nourish the heart, moisten the kidney, tranquilize the spirit, and calm the mind."

Since there are many traditional Chinese medical herbs that can calm the heart and tranquilize the mind, why do I specifically mention the platycladi seed? First, the platycladi seed is mild in nature and will not hurt the body even if taken over a long period of time. This is also why it is considered as a top-grade medicine in the *Materia Medica of Shennong*. Further, because the cypress seed contains volatile oil, a pillow filled with it gives out fragrance and invigorates the mind.

This method is particularly effective to mental workers and overanxious people. You can also use it if you are under a great deal of pressure or lack sobriety. If you cannot find cypress seeds near your home, you can buy some in a TCM pharmacy to make this sort of pillow.

Similarly, many people, when they feel depressed, like to take a walk along a riverbank lined on both sides with willows, which will immediately cheer them up. This is because the willow can clear away heat and ease pain.

In addition, the poplar tree is effective in warming the organs. If you are physically weak and fall sick constantly, you can exercise in a poplar forest.

4. Going to Bed Before 11 PM and Taking a Nap at Noon

For many years, I have maintained the habit, no matter how busy I am, of sparing 20 minutes at midday to close my eyes for meditation. As short as this meditation is, I feel vigorous and energetic after each session. I lecture the whole morning, but only need 20 minutes at noon to regain vigor and energy in the afternoon. By contrast, the young people listening to my afternoon lecture often look tired and absent-minded.

Ancient Chinese people have realized the importance of an early night's sleep and a noontime nap. From 11 p.m. to 1 a.m., the yin energy is at its height, while the yang energy is waning. Mice are connected to yin and are thus most active in this period. But humans often work in the daytime and need yang energy to aid them. Therefore, they should finish their work and go to bed before 11 p.m., because by then, their yang energy has become insufficient. The best way to preserve the yang energy during this period is through sound sleep, which will ensure that one can engage in work in high spirits the following morning. On the other hand, from 11 a.m. to 1 p.m., the yang energy is at its peak, while the yin energy is waning. According to the *Inner Canon of the Yellow Emperor*, an ancient Chinese medical text, "One should sleep when the yang energy runs out and awake when the yin energy goes to its end." An early sleep can nourish the kidneys, and a noontime nap nourishes the heart. Therefore, a proper rest during these two periods benefits not only yin and yang, but also the coordination between the heart and kidney. It enables the internal heat to go down and the kidney water to rise. The more coordination between the heart and kidney, the better the spirits will be. For all these years, alongside going to bed early, I have persevered in meditating every day at noon. I close my eyes and think about nothing. At the same time, I put my tongue against my palate and swallow my saliva, imagining the saliva is going down to the kidney. If I feel too exhausted and cannot make up for the energy lost through meditation, I also take a midday nap, from which I always awake reinvigorated.

On average, a person needs 8 hours of sleep a day, but the most important periods are the 4 hours from 11 p.m. to 1 a.m. and from 11 a.m. to 1 p.m.

Many friends complain to me that they suffer from insomnia. One was a business tycoon. She was very busy and did not often go to bed until early morning. Even when she was in bed, she could not fall asleep, but was always thinking about her contracts and her company. Gradually, her body rebelled. At first, she was in low spirits and dizzy during the day. Later, she started to have menstrual disorders and spots began to appear on her face. When she came to my lectures, she complained to me that it was not that she did not sleep well, but that she could not fall asleep at all. When she did go to bed early, she would toss and turn, lost in various worries and conjectures.

In fact, many people suffer from insomnia because of anxiety. What they do not know is that the day and night represent yin and yang in nature, and many things should be done in the day because it is the time for movement, when yang energy grows and prospers. By contrast, night is for quiet time and rest, when yang energy declines and yin energy prospers. Therefore, at night, we should put down whatever work we have at hand and have a good rest, if we hope to avoid physical problems. It is important to keep in mind that only with a good rest at night can we work better the next day.

I told her that the reason for her insomnia was that she was physically in bed, but mentally elsewhere. If she hoped to fall asleep quickly, she needed to calm her mind first and try not to think of anything. She might try pressing her legs together while sitting on the bed to meditation. The method I recommended was to: Sit cross-legged in a natural position, overlap the hands and place them on the legs, breathe evenly until you feel the pores open and close with each breath, and finally lie down to sleep as soon as you feel drowsy.

Another simple method in Zen medicine that helps one sleep is to try to imagine that your body is totally relaxed, like sugar melting in water. The big toe melts first, then the other toes, then the legs, then the thighs, and soon all the way up the body. By the time the whole body is melted, you will naturally be asleep already.

Modern people are often physically and mentally exhausted. They seldom have time to sleep early or take a midday nap. Consequently, they are tortured by sub-optimal health, which affects their work and life. We should make full use of the two prime periods to rest and nourish our kidneys and hearts.

5. Achieving Balance between Yin and Yang

Yin and yang are the conception of nature summarized by ancient Chinese thinkers. In this system of thought, the heaven is yang, and the earth is yin. Yin exists in yang, and yang also exists in yin. The energy of the heavens descends and moves on the earth, and the energy of the earth ascends into the heavens. It is the balance between yin and yang that gives birth to the world we live in, which is reflected in the sun and the moon, the day and the night, summer and winter, and other similar pairs of opposites.

Just as the imbalance between yin and yang on earth will cause natural disasters, so the imbalance in our bodies will cause disease. Those whose yin and yang are balanced have strong vitality and psychological endurance. They eat well, sleep well, and look great. They are happy and spirited, and they enjoy a strong capacity for dealing with emergencies, great adaptability, good stamina, and strong resistance to disease. By contrast, those whose yin and yang are imbalanced are prone to illness.

What is the yang energy? It is what is superficial, upward, hyperactive, intensive, clear, and light. Insufficient yang energy will result in the failure of certain internal organs, causing cold limbs, weak breath, waning strength, fatigue, a weak pulse, and other similar conditions. Where do we find yang energy? The sun. When we lack yang energy, we should gather it in sunny places on fine days. At sunrise, we can take deep breaths as we face the sun, and the yang energy can enter our bodies through our nostrils and pores. Between 11 a.m. to 1 p.m., we can nourish yang energy either through sleep, repose, or meditation for 15 to 30 minutes. The best posture is to recline or lie on the back. When it is cold, we should bask ourselves in the sun, which will effectively supplement our yang energy and make us healthier. We can also eat more warm foods, such as Chinese leeks or walnut kernels. In addition, many seasonings can increase the yang energy, such as ginger or aniseeds. If we feel our yang energy is insufficient, we can add these seasonings into the dishes we cook.

When we have been sick for a long time or when we are excessively tired, our yin energy may become insufficient and there may be surplus of yang energy in us. As a result, we may suffer from excessive internal heat. When this is the case, we can take a walk under the moon after supper, which effectively nourishes the yin energy. We can also take time to regularly travel in mountain forests, or by rivers and lakes, which not only nourishes the yin energy, but also improves our mood. Foods that improve the yin energy are plentiful, including tremella, lily bulb, and pears.

As long as we can maintain the balance between yin and yang, we can live a longer, healthier life.

6. The Shaolin Breath-Holding Technique

The Shaolin breath-holding technique is often mentioned in Chinese martial arts novels. It is, in fact, very simple, consisting of holding your breath after each inhalation and exhalation.

Hold your breath after inhaling: If you are physically weak, you can try this method. The reason is that this method extends the time of inhalation, which can improve your body's capacity for stress by stimulating the sympathetic nerve. It is like giving yourself an extra boost of energy, and you will naturally feel vigorous and stronger.

Exhale before holding your breath: This extends the time of exhalation, which can sustain your body through stimulating the parasympathetic nerve. It also helps clear away deficient heat. If you feel fidgety and worried, you may try this method. If you feel a lack of strength or spirit, you may try the previous method.

One of the methods to practice the breath-holding technique is to sit with your legs crossed in a natural position. The steps are to first sit with your legs crossed, the arches of the feet facing backwards. (A female practitioner should bend her left leg, with the left heel in alignment with the Huiyin point and the right foot touching the left lower leg. A male practitioner should have his right heel in alignment with the Huiyin point and his left foot touching the right lower leg.) Then, overlap your hands as shown in the figure and put them on your legs. In this position, practice abdominal breathing. Finally, after these steps are completed, rub your palms and face and pat your body all over to relax.

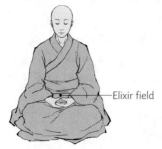

Elixir field

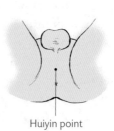

Huiyin point

7. Countering Illness with Willpower

Willpower is released from the energy field of humans by way of the brain. Humans are the combination of two matters, yin and yang, and these matters have energy. The energy released in the process of thinking is known as willpower.

Willpower is of great benefit to our bodies, and training our willpower regularly is a method of health preservation. Let's use breathing to illustrate the training of our willpower. First, keep yourself from distractions and relax your body, then inhale deeply and try to imagine the circulation of energy and blood. Finally, exhale and try to imagine their back-flow. In fact, energy and blood circulation is always there, but it is only when it coordinates with your willpower that it can generate greater effects. Without you realizing it, this process makes your body and heart more robust.

In addition to this breathing exercise, there are many other exercises can be done to effectively use willpower, such as acupressure massage and functional recovery trainings. When you massage your vital points, use your willpower to think from which channel the massage takes effect. When you exercise, try to think which part of your body or which internal organ is strengthened by a certain action. The unity of the heart and action produces greater healing effects.

Willpower is a very powerful energy field that can be strengthened by reduced desires, a peaceful state of mind, and doing good deeds. In other words, moral integrity is the source of the energy field. The more concentrated the willpower, the more powerful the field.

All a person's desires are determined by the heart, which is the organ that generates desire. Therefore, humans' energy fields are controlled by the heart. The more desire the heart generates, the more scattered the energy field is, the smaller its impact on the outside world, and the weaker its ability to protect itself.

On the other hand, the fewer the desires of the heart, the more condensed the energy field becomes, the bigger impact it has on the outside world, and the stronger its ability to protect itself.

When you live a simple, selfless, and peaceful life, your energy field is at its most powerful, and its power to resist external aggressions reaches its peak. This is called the realm of Dhyana in Zen Buddhism. The willpower one releases at this moment often produces incredible effects. If you wish to have a strong physique, this method is worth trying.

8. Sleeping in a Warm Environment

Many people have cold limbs. They do not feel warm in winter, no matter how thick their blanket is. When they ask me for a solution, I tell them there are two methods. One is to soak the feet in warm water for 30 minutes, and the other is to generate a light sweat by exercising 30 minutes each night before going to bed. They can choose either of these methods.

Their feedback after a week is always, "Now it is warm under the blanket and the problem of getting cold limbs while I sleep is gone."

I ask them, "Do you know why the problem is gone?"

"Yes," they say, "after soaking my feet in warm water or exercising for 30 minutes, I feel warm all over. When I'm under the blanket, I warm the blanket first, then it warms me."

This is not only the way to good health, but also to a good life. If we can help others to have warmth first, others will help us in return if we are in trouble.

9. Maintaining Childlike Innocence

Many people feel that the hospital is overcrowded today, but in fact, it was the same when I began to work in a hospital in the 1960s. At that time, there were fewer patients, but also fewer hospitals and doctors. Therefore, just like their counterparts today, doctors in those days would remain busy for the whole day, from the time they started work in the morning.

One day when I was terribly busy, I felt dizzy and fidgety. To adjust my mood, I held a cup of water and stood by the window to stare at the green trees outside.

On the balcony was a pot of roses I had placed there. By then, all the flowers were in bloom, a dozen of which were big and beautiful. I started to appreciate the roses. With childlike innocence, I began to count the number of flower petals and layers. I became fascinated and did not come to myself until I had been called several times. When I did come to myself, I found, to my surprise, that I was no longer fidgety.

Realizing that this was a good method, of relaxing, in the following days, whenever I was extremely busy with work, I would spare some time to count the flower petals. As time passed, I no longer needed to stare at the flowers. As long as I closed my eyes, roses would pop into my mind. I felt as if I were in a sea of roses, relaxed and happy.

Later, I seldom felt fidgety. I often used this method of counting flower petals when I worked in the hospital. Once, I noticed a scene in a TV program. A mom was counting stars with her young child, who muttered one, two, three, four, and so on. Often, the child got mixed up and start to count again. Suddenly, I realized, "Isn't it the same as my counting flower petals?"

When childlike innocence is evoked in a person, they will certainly grow happy and calm.

10. Relieving Fatigue through Poetry and Meditating

I often worked more than 16 hours a day when I was a doctor. In addition, I also had to regularly give emergency treatment to patients. However, I never felt exhausted. This had a great deal to do with my unique method of relieving fatigue.

When I entered the Shaolin Temple in childhood, my master taught me a poem composed by the Tang poet Wang Wei (701–761):

An Autumn Evening in My Villa
In the empty mountains, fresh after a shower,
Autumn thickens with oncoming dusk—
Tranquil moonlight glistens among pines,
And crystal water bubbles over the pebbles.

According to my master, when you feel tired after exercising, reading, or doing manual work, you should find a tranquil place to recite this poem. While reading, try to imagine that you are in this mountain forest. After a shower, the mountain and valleys are quieter and more secluded. When night falls, the breeze rises, making you feel the thickening of autumn. The bright moon casts down its light through the leaves of the pine trees and the crystal water is bubbling through the rocks and over the pebbles.

Alternatively, you can take a book, close your eyes, and recite this poem as you shake your head. Of course, what is important is that you can try to recall the scene created in this poem in your mind while reading, giving full play to your imagination. As time goes on, when you think of this poem, you will immediately feel as if you were part of the scene, and your annoyance and fatigue will soon disappear.

11. Practicing Mental Suggestion

It has been 20 years since I was diagnosed with terminal colon cancer in 1996, but I am still alive, and my health is improving. Aged as I am, I am still as spirited as a young person. I remember that when I was hospitalized, many well-known doctors came to visit me and gave me their diagnoses. It was not until recently that I knew that, after reading my medical report, many of them believed that I could not possibly survive the disease.

Many people asked me later, "How did you pull through?"

"Do you believe I have a powerful army to help me?" I replied.

They were all confused. But "a powerful army" was a mental

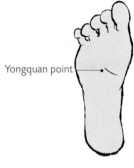

Yongquan point

suggestion. Every day, after practicing *Ba Duan Jin* and taking a happy walk (see page 90), I would sit on the bed (initially I lay on the bed), close my eyes, and do breathing exercise. I would then start mental suggestions. All my white cells, phagocytes, and major immune systems are now ready to launch an attack. They are waiting for the brain to give orders. As soon as the order is given, they, like soldiers in a powerful army, will kill the cancer cells one by one, using swords or spears. Then I would imagine myself exhaling deeply, discharging the dead cells to the ground through the Yongquan point. Layers and layers of cancer cells were killed with the repeated attacks of these soldiers.

Superficially, I did not move a muscle, but I became boiling hot, even slightly sweaty, after each attempt. At the same time, I grew more spirited and was gradually recovering from the illness with each passing day.

In fact, what cancer fears is the human immune system. Although this method is a suggestive therapy, it has a significant medical effect, as it mobilizes the yang energy in the body and enables the immune system to play its role. I know many cancer patients who have recovered due to their successful mobilization of the yang energy in their bodies.

If you fall sick, you can use this sort of suggestive therapy. When you have mobilized your entire immune system, you will become extremely tenacious. Then, what does it matter if you have a few little cancer cells?

12. Simple Food Therapies

Three White Ingredients

According to the ancients, heaven has three treasures, the sun, the moon, and the stars, and the earth has three treasures, water, fire, and wind. A human similarly has three treasures, the essence of life, vital energy, and spirit. This means that the essence of life, vital energy, and spirit are crucial to our state of life, and as long as we have enough of them, we will naturally be healthy and have a long life. We must be careful if we feel languished, short of breath, or physically weak.

Recently, a new volunteer worker from a wealthy family came to the Temple. She said that she volunteered to work for the Buddha because, on the one hand, she was bored at home, having nothing to do, and on the other, she hoped that by doing volunteer work, she would bring blessings to her family. She was only two years older than me, but had suffered from high blood pressure and hyperlipemia. Her mental condition was very poor, and so was her physical condition. She did not even have the strength to climb to the third floor of a building, and she would doze off after each meal. Judging from the perspective of the traditional Chinese medicine, she lacked the three treasures essential to human beings, that is, the essence of life, vital energy, and spirit.

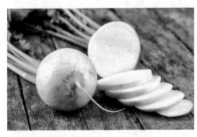

White turnips.

Based on her condition, I recommended for her diet the three white ingredients, rice, salt, and white turnips.

Bland and mild, rice invigorates the spleen and stomach, benefits the essence of life, and enhances the memory. The white turnip can improve the immunity of the body, promote digestion, help gastrointestinal motility, increase metabolism, and, most importantly, conserve vital energy. As an indispensable condiment in daily life, salt can spur the kidney's energy, which is the primary force to maintain life. It is only when one eats enough salt that he will have strength.

If a meal contains the three white ingredients, it can replenish the essence of life, vital energy, and spirit. According to *Valuable Prescriptions for Emergencies*, a classic book of medicine in ancient China, "One should not eat or drink excessively. The elderly cannot digest well if they over-indulge in food and drink, as their spleen and stomach have thinner skins." Instead of having too much meat, old people would be better off eating more meals containing the three white ingredients. In addition, one should not be too particular about the exact proportion of each of the ingredients in food, but should use them as we sees fit.

A month later, the woman told me that she was lighter and stronger. After two more months, she was a different person from when she first came.

Triple White Porridge

Many people feel puzzled about why monks who eat vegetarian food are healthy and fit, while the health of those who enjoy fine food every day has completely broken down.

The temple I live in is at the foot of a mountain, which is less than 1,000 meters high. After offering incense to Buddha, many pilgrims will try to climb the mountain. However, most of them gasp for breath as they climb and are unable to reach the mountaintop without several rests. By contrast, the younger monks in the temple and I will go up and down the mountain several times each day, feeling not the least bit tired. Why are we so energetic? It has much to do with the porridge we eat at each meal.

Porridge can enhance the physical strength of the one who eats it. An old gentleman once came to me for medical treatment. He was a man with yin deficiency and heat hyperactivity, and he was often thirsty and fidgety. He did not pass much urine, and what he did was very yellow. He felt heat radiating from inside his bones, causing him vexation and insomnia. During the hot summer, he would sweat profusely, as if sitting in a sauna. In addition, since there was heat in his heart and spleen, his digestive system was not good either. He had difficulty digesting greasy and dry food, and he felt full all the time.

I asked him to eat rice porridge every morning and evening, because rice can ease the spleen and stomach, nourish yin, moisten the respiratory tract, get rid of irritation and thirst, and act as a diuretic. If added with some white poria, which helps urination, and white haricot beans, which remove summer heat and dampness, the porridge will have an even greater healing effect. Moreover, with white poria, the porridge can not only ease frustration and nourish the spleen and stomach, but it will also calm the heart, tranquilize the mind, and help maintain a good complexion.

I happened to find this porridge prescription in a medical book. It is particularly suited to physically weak people, as it can make them feel energetic, ease their sense of hunger and thirst, and ultimately help them live longer. Since the three ingredients the porridge contains are all white, it is named the triple white porridge. The recipe is as follows:

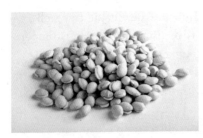

White haricot beans.

Ingredients: White poria (20 g), white haricot beans (60 g), and rice (100 g).

Cooking method: Cook over a high heat until the porridge is done, then over a low heat for another 40 minutes.

After eating the porridge for a month, the old man's health had improved greatly. He felt much happier and did not get fidgety as easily as he had before. His digestion was getting better, and his cheeks were much rosier. A physical check-up in the hospital showed that every index had improved under this diet.

Triple Black Porridge

Eyes are the door of wisdom and the window of the soul. It is through the eyes that people discern things and increase their knowledge. Buddhists depend on their eyes to read Buddhist scriptures and learn about the universe. A highly cultivated Buddhist possesses bright eyes, as well as the eyes of the heart, which help him understand more deeply the causes behind all matters. In this sense, the eyes are crucial to a Buddhist.

Ms. Zhu recently had some trouble with her eyes. She could not see clearly, as if a layer of gauze covered her eyes, and she often saw stars. When she consulted me for her illness, I knew immediately that the cause was poor eye nutrition resulting from a deficiency in the liver and kidney and the failure of the vital energy and blood to travel to her eyes.

I recommended her the triple black porridge that contains black sesame seeds, black beans, and black rice. It is thus named because both the ingredients and the porridge they produce are black. The recipe is as follows:

Ingredients: Black sesame seeds (20 g), black beans (20 g), and black rice (20 g).

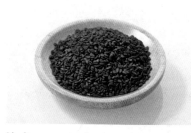

Cooking method: First, roast the black sesame seeds and black beans, then grind them into powder. Wash the black rice clean. Then, cook the rice over a medium heat until it is done. Finally, add the powder into the porridge and continue to boil until the whole mixture is thoroughly cooked.

Black sesame seeds.

According to traditional Chinese medicine, black food nourishes the kidney, the condition of which is closely associated with that of eyes. Bland and mild, sesame seeds benefit yin and moisten the respiratory tract. Black beans are bland and warm, capable of nourishing yin, reinforcing the kidney, replenishing blood, and improving eyesight. This porridge is particularly effective for those who have a poor eyesight due to a deficiency in the liver and kidney, because it helps blood circulation, moistens the skin, nourishes the liver and kidney, and improves eyesight. Moreover, the porridge is also very effective in invigorating the brain and improving hearing.

For two weeks, Ms. Zhu had been eating this porridge in the morning and at night. As a result, her eyesight improved and she could see clearly.

I once had a friend who was 62 and very forgetful. What's worse, his hearing was poor, too, and thus he made a fool of himself on many occasions. He liked to play cards, but often made mistakes due to his poor hearing. He often felt a cicada was chirping in his ears. Consequently, he got angry with himself at the end of each game. But after eating this black porridge for some time, his tinnitus was gone, and he was no longer forgetful.

According to traditional Chinese medicine, the liver and kidney have a common source. When we are old, our livers and kidneys degenerate and do not operate as efficiently as they used to. When this occurs, we should replenish them with this sweet, delicious black porridge.

13. A Cup of Lukewarm Water

Many people who exercise daily still have a poor health. This might have to do with either their method of exercising or their incorrect habits.

Some people will go to bed covered with sweat as soon as they finish exercising. This does harm to their health because they have failed to replenish their bodies with water when it is needed. Others will belt down cold water the moment they finish exercising, not knowing that cold drinks may impair their stomach and their health.

Whatever exercise I do, whether it is meditating, walking,

or practicing martial arts, I will place a cup of boiled water beside me before the exercise begins. After the exercise, which usually lasts about 45 minutes, the water has cooled down to about 30 degrees. I will then drink it slowly. This not only makes me feel comfortable, but also meets my body's needs.

Why do I advocate drinking lukewarm water? Because it balances the yin and yang energies in our bodies. Doing exercise increases yang energy, while drinking lukewarm water nourishes yin and generates body fluids, as lukewarm water is connected to yin energy. In addition, according to Western medicine, water should be supplemented after exercising.

To make exercise more effective, we should start with a cup of lukewarm water.

14. Relaxation Exercise

Doing acupuncture, I often come across patients who are rigid all over due to fear. I pat them on the shoulders and tell them to relax, because, otherwise, I cannot get the needles into their flesh.

This kind of tension is visible, but today, many people live with invisible tension. For example, working long hours in a high pressure environment and at a fast pace, people may suffer from muscular soreness, insomnia, dizziness, and listlessness. These symptoms are the same as those that appear in an acupuncture treatment.

A relaxation exercise in the Shaolin Temple is good for such cases, as it can eliminate tension in the mind, internal organs, and muscles. This exercise is very simple, and it can be done in a standing, sitting, or lying posture, with the sitting posture being the best. You can also adjust the posture based on your own habits or health condition.

The Standing Posture
Stand facing the front, with your feet shoulder-width apart and

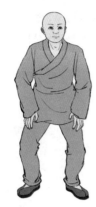

your arms hanging in a natural position at your sides. Put your hands against the thighs, tuck your belly in, lower the head slightly, tuck your lower jaw inward, keep your backbone straight, keep your eyes slightly closed, and press your tongue against the palate.

The Sitting Posture

Sit on a stool of appropriate height, knees bent at 90 degrees with 20 cm between them, backbone straight, and lower jaw tucked inward. Make sure the Baihui point and the Huiyin point form a straight line. Put your hands naturally on your thighs, palms down, press your tongue against the palate, and keep your eyes slightly closed.

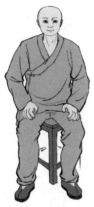

The Lying Posture

Lying on the side: Lie on your side in a soft bed. Adjust the height of the pillow until your neck vertebra are kept straight. Straighten one leg on the bed and bend the other leg in a natural position. Place your hand above and in front of the body, palm down. Place your other hand below on the pillow horizontally, palm facing up. Lying on either side is fine, but it is suggested that heart disease patients lie on the right side.

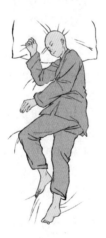

Lying on the back: Lie on the back in a natural position. Adjust the pillow until you feel comfortable. Straighten your legs and put your feet together in a natural position. Place the arms on both sides of

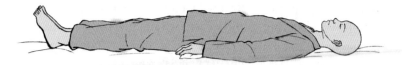

the body, palms down. Hold the tongue against the palate and lightly close your eyes.

The exercise is very simple, involving relaxation from head to toe. Specifically, you should try to relax from your head, face, neck, shoulders, upper arm, elbow, forearm, hands, chests, back, waist, hip, thighs, knees, calves, and finally to the feet.

Breathe one to three times as you relax each of the body part. Breathe in as you like, but when breathing out, you should consciously relax the relevant body part, each in sequence. If you have difficulty breathing properly, you can wait until you have familiarized yourself with the order of relaxation. There is no need to do the relaxation exercise too frequently. Three times a day is enough.

You can try this exercise as often as you feel sluggish or mentally stressed due to pressure at work. In other words, it is fit for those who are troubled by sub-optimal health.

15. Shaolin Standing Exercise

Many people do not know what *qi* is. It is in fact the spirit. The body is the basis of life, and the spirit is its distillation.

By way of analogy, we note that a cup is used to contain water. As a container, it serves its contents. However, if something is wrong with the container, the contents will leak. The same is true of a human being. If he is in poor health, his spirit and energy will gradually dissipate, and as a result, he will look dispirited. In modern society, the huge pressure and the ignorance of health preservation lead many people to overspend their energy. They look weak even when they are young.

The Shaolin Temple has a standing exercise for internal

adjustments. Characterized by the cultivation of both the body and spirit and an association of activity and inertia, it is a basic technique for Shaolin warrior-monks to develop and replenish internal energy after practicing martial arts.

This exercise can keep the muscles all over the body in constant static tension, thereby harmonizing energy and blood and promoting physiological metabolism. Practicing this technique regularly over a long period will make you energetic and vigorous, increase the smooth flow of energy and blood, benefit health, and prevent disease. The exercise is highly effective for those who are troubled with chronic diseases, physical weakness, and poor health. The method is laid out systematically here.

Preparational Movements

Stand facing the front with your feet shoulder-width apart, your arms hanging down in a natural position, and your hands laid lightly against the thighs. Keep your body and the neck vertebra straight, the lower jaw slightly back, and the eyes looking straight in front. Relax and try to imagine that the yang energy of the sun enters your body through the Baihui point and the yin energy of the earth enters through the Yongquan point. They

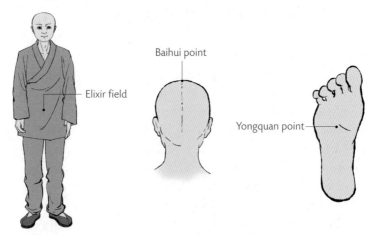

Baihui point

Elixir field

Yongquan point

will converge at the elixir field and integrate with your own vital energy. This is known as the "unity of heaven, earth, and man." Maintain this state as you breathe ten times.

Regular Movements

Move the left foot half a step to the left, putting a distance between the feet that is three times the length of the foot. Imagine that your feet are rooted deeply into the ground like a big tree. Bend your knees and do a half squat, as if riding a horse. (Beginners don't need to push themselves too hard and so can squat a little bit higher.) Meanwhile, raise your arms slowly to shoulder height and turn the hands into a sword-shaped posture, palms down, fingertips forward, and hands shoulder width apart. Keep the upper body upright, hold in the stomach slightly, straighten the head and neck, tuck in the lower jaw, and keep the Baihui point, Huiyin point, and the central point between the heels on a straight line. Bend the knees outward in a natural position, keeping them in a straight line with the toes. Look straight ahead, eyes slightly closed, and breathe naturally. Remain in this standing posture for 20–40 minutes each time.

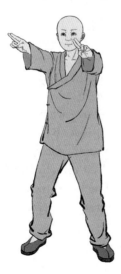

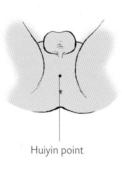

Huiyin point

Concluding Movements

Withdraw the hands and stand upright. Breathe 10 times with your hands overlapped on your abdomen. Rub your hands, face, and neck and the Dazhui point (the most prominent joint on the back of your neck when your lower your head). Then, move the left foot half a step to the left and do a half squat. Put your hands on your thighs, fingertips facing each other, and circle the legs six times from the outside inward, then from the inside out. After that, put your feet together, squat with your hands on your thighs, and circle the legs six times to the left, then six times to the right. Straighten up and pat your body all over from top to bottom, the left hand patting the right side of the body and the right hand patting the left side. This will get rid of the soreness you might feel when you practice this standing exercise.

In the beginning, your legs and arms may ache or shake. This is normal. You need to persevere with the exercise. However, if you feel dizzy, sick, or flustered, stop at once and wait until you have fully recovered.

16. Taking a "Happy Walk" after Each Meal

An old Chinese saying notes, "Walk a hundred steps after each meal and you will live a long life." As for me, I often walk about 30 to 40 minutes after each of my three meals. However, unlike others, I take a "happy walk" that is typical of the Shaolin Temple.

"Happy walk," as the name suggests, can make people who walk happy. In fact, the exercise was created by earlier monks as a way of preserving health and treating disease. Based on Buddhist principles and the six-word breathing technique (see page 60) mentioned above, the "happy walk" it can effectively invigorate one's health, improve immune functions, promote lesion absorption, clear away heat, purge intense heat, tone deficiencies, and enhance kidney function.

The "happy walk" can either be slow or fast. Its method of practice is outlined here.

Slow Walk

By taking a slow walk, you control the number of steps you take to 8 to 20 a minute. But here, one step includes moving forward with your right foot and left foot one time each. Unlike taking a usual walk, before moving a step forward, you need to touch the ground with your big toe, raise your heel, and slightly move the heel towards the inside. And your body should also follow the heel to move, but in an opposite direction. For example, when you move the right heel towards the inside (or the left), your body should twist towards the right. Pay attention that you do not twist your heel or body too much.

In addition, do not overswing your hands. They should move close to the abdominal midline or between the stomach and groin in a natural way, with the palms facing the stomach.

The exercise aims at stimulating the liver and spleen meridians (see page 142), which start from the big toe, one on its inside and the other on its outside. The liver meridian, once stimulated, can relax the liver, remove depression, and make you feel happy, and hence the designation "happy walk." Since you often take a walk after meals, the spleen meridian, once stimulated, can help you digest and tone your spleen.

Fast Walk

A fast walk is the same as a slow walk, but the frequency is raised to 30 to 60 steps a minute. You can choose either one, based on your physical condition.

Breathing

What deserves attention is that the happy walk must be supplemented with some breathing techniques.

The first method involves two inhalations followed by one exhalation. It means completing the inhalation in two steps and the exhalation in one step. For example, inhale when you move forward, first with your left and then your right foot, and exhale when you move your left foot again. This method is fit for those who are physically weak.

The second method involves one inhalation and two exhalations. It means completing the inhalation in one step and the exhalation in two steps. This method is fit for excess-syndrome patients, such as those who suffer from lung heat, excessive internal heat, agitation, and a burning sensation in the five centers.

The third method involves an inhalation and an exhalation. It means completing the inhalation in one step and the exhalation in another step. This method is very effective if you do it after recovery from an illness.

My grandpa lived a vagrant's life, but he did not die until he was 97. This had much to do with the happy walk he took every day. As a child, I was happy when I saw him take a happy walk free and easy.

17. The Day's Plan Starts with an Early Morning

In ancient China, both officials and the ordinary people had to get up very early in the morning. They would be laughed at and considered as lazy by their neighbors if they failed to rise with the cock's crow. Even the emperor was no exception. For example, the three emperors of the Qing dynasty, Kangxi (1654–1722), Yongzheng (1678–1735), and Qianlong (1711–1799), often got up at 3 a.m. to prepare for their morning duties. They would finish all official business by 5 a.m.

It has been a time-honored rule for monks in temples to retire at the evening drumbeat and rise at the morning bell to do their morning lessons at 4 a.m. Morning hours are the best time of the day to work, and they are also the time that yang energy occurs. It is wise for us to get up early to work as well.

From the medical point of view, from 3 to 5 o'clock in the morning is the time the lung meridian works. Rising at this time will extend lung energy, help metabolism, lower turbid energy, and promote yang energy. From 5 to 7 o'clock is the time the large intestine meridian is prosperous, and it is the time for the body to have a thorough cleanup, meaning that the large intestine meridian needs to discharge the metabolite processed in the lung meridian out of the body. If we stay in bed during this time, our large intestines will not get enough exercise and the discharge cannot be properly done. As a result, the metabolite will remain in our body, endangering our blood, internal organs, and bones. From 7 to 9 o'clock is the time the stomach meridian thrives. Since the intestines and stomach work best during this time, we should get up and have breakfast then. If we do not get up by then, the gastric acid we secrete will severely erode our gastric mucosa, causing intestinal tract diseases.

However, very few modern people get up before 6 a.m. Many work and rest irregularly, staying up all night and waking up in the morning without an alarm. They are asleep when the lung meridian works, and they are still in sleep when the large intestine meridian and the stomach meridian work. Why do people who are reluctant to get up in the morning feel that the more they sleep, the more tired they become? It is because they sleep at the wrong times. Although they sleep for long periods, they are out of spirits the whole day.

Refusing to get up in the morning is against the law of nature. It is also a kind of laziness. Only when we follow the law of nature can we become healthy and successful.

Chapter IV
Curing Physical Illness with Zen Medicine

1. The Digestive System

There are many disease of the digestive system, including pathological changes in the esophagus, stomach, colon, and bowels. They have a high morbidity rate and seriously affect one's eating patterns. But without taking in food, we cannot supplement the nutrition to our bodies, which will impair our ability to resist disease.

A rule in Buddhism is "no food after midday." Therefore, a Buddhist does not usually take in food after noon, or they will violate this discipline. When I was very young, my master often warned me that food eaten in the evening could not be digested and would cause health problems.

Our internal organs also have their own schedules. For example, the stomach works best between 7 and 9 a.m., and food taken during this period can be easily digested and absorbed. The afternoon is the rest time for the intestines and stomach. Therefore, the Buddha instructs us that we should drink pure water in the afternoon to dilute what we ate in the morning. This will help our body excrete and absorb, and it will refresh our internal organs. However, many modern people have the habit of going to bed late and getting up late. As a result, the stomach is empty in the morning when it needs to take in the essence of nature, but stuffed with abundant fish and meat at night when it needs to rest. Since the regular schedule of our internal organs is broken, we are prone to disease.

An old Chinese saying suggests that if we eat less at supper, we will enjoy a longer life, because many diseases are the result of overeating in the evening. According to modern medicine, our metabolism starts up at 4:00 in the morning and reaches its peak at 4:00 in the afternoon. Therefore, the best time for us to add nutrition to our body is at breakfast and lunch times. After 4:00 p.m., our metabolism begins to slow down, making it difficult to digest food, allowing it to turn to fat instead.

The Buddhist rule of no food after midday is not meant to conserve grain, but to rid people of the three evils in their hearts, greediness, anger, and ignorance. If we hanker after material comfort, our spiritual growth will be hindered and our body destroyed. We will not starve if we skip supper, but we can die from overeating at supper. Therefore, for health's sake, please carefully consider this rule.

Insufficient Gastric Motility

I do not prefer luxurious food. I need only a hardened steamed bun to satisfy my hunger. I do not drink any water, either. People who hear this are often dumbfounded, asking me whether my stomach can bear this diet. I smile and tell them, "Hardened as the bun is, it stimulates the stomach, which secretes more gastric juice and enhances gastric motility."

Our organs have inertia. If we do not use them, they will gradually deteriorate. Fine food tastes soft and good, but our intestines and stomach will become slack with these foods, because they do not need to take pains to secrete digestive juice. Therefore, people who wine and dine every day are apt to stomach ailments.

I once came across a benefactor with stomach troubles. He was extremely particular about eating. His food must be crispy and soft, and easily swallowed with little chewing. However, his stomach illness did not improve, but instead grew more serious. I told him that food is digested by gastric juices, and if there is too much water in the food, the stomach will not produce more gastric juices. In consequence, the deterioration of the stomach function will lead stomach troubles to become even more serious.

Later, I suggested that he eat hardened streamed buns. If the bun was too cold, it could be warmed in an oven for one minute, making it crispy so that it would activate the stomach. Omeprazole (OME), a stomach medicine, serves to inhibit the secretion of gastric acid, since many stomach troubles, such as stomachaches, regurgitation, and burning sensations in the stomach are all caused by over-secretion of gastric acid. Hardened buns have the same effect, neutralizing excess gastric acid. For this reason, long-term stomach patients can eat more of these buns. Instead of swallowing the bread, they should chew each bite dozens of times so that more saliva will be secreted. According to traditional Chinese medicine, saliva shares a source with blood, making it quite valuable for its ability to generate blood and make people more vigorous and energetic.

Moreover, chewing hardened buns can also strengthen the teeth, because it increases the chances for the upper teeth to meet the lower teeth, which is a traditional Chinese toothcare exercise. Doctors of the traditional Chinese medicine believe that teeth reflect the condition of the kidney, so strengthening the teeth is a way of toning the kidneys.

Finally, the more we chew hardened buns, the stronger the digestive function of our spleen and stomach will be, and the healthier we will become.

Seven years ago, I told this method to an elderly man whose teeth had loosened, I asked him to stick with it for a while. Now, at 75, his teeth are still healthy, and so is his body. As simple as it is, this method is very effective, and we are sure to benefit from it if we persevere.

Gastric Distension
According to Buddhist scriptures, we are born to suffer. But

heaven's way is cyclical, and after suffering comes happiness. Therefore, we must learn to adapt to sufferings and forge ourselves through them. If we only think of our stomachs and fail to live a disciplined life, we will eventually become ill.

For example, we all know that illness finds its way into the body through the mouth, but how many of us can resist the temptation of fine food? Once a tycoon told me that he had come down with stomach troubles and cholecystitis. He felt full, and he had a bitter taste in the mouth. When I asked him about his appetite, he said that he had previously had a great appetite and drank a lot of alcohol, but now his appetite was gone.

He was surprised when I told him that his loss of appetite was due to his previous overeating.

"It's simple," I explained. "You ate too much, which has enlarged your stomach. Therefore, you need bile to digest what you ate. You have a bitter taste in the mouth and cholecystitis, because the bile you secreted is excessive. In addition, when you got drunk, you would get up very late in the morning. By skipping breakfast, the bile your body produced in the morning could do nothing but irritate your stomach. That's why you have lost your appetite and have a bitter taste in the mouth."

Then I told him that all his stomach troubles would be cured if he would eat only something that "tasted bad." The recipe was simple. After cleaning an onion and bitter gourd, I instructed him to soak them in water for three to four minutes, then eat them.

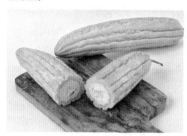
Bitter gourd.

With its bitterness, the bitter gourd would lower the concentration of glucose in the blood. However, as it is cool in nature, it will hurt the spleen and stomach if eaten too frequently. Onion is used as a balance to drive away cold, stimulate secretion of the stomach, intestines, and digestive glands, increase the appetite, improve digestion, and remove gastric distension. The patient followed my advice, eating onion and bitter gourd at each meal and refraining from eating meat. A month later, both his stomach trouble and his cholecystitis were gone.

Digestive Tract Diseases

When I was a doctor, I once came across a patient who came to the hospital for a checkup. He was diagnosed with esophagus cancer and was immediately hospitalized. When I visited the ward, I found him extremely emaciated and terrified. I asked him, "How did you come to the hospital?"

"On foot," he answered.

Then I replied, "Since you still have the strength to walk, your illness is not as serious as you think."

After hearing my diagnosis, he finally regained some vigor. I urged him to take medicine on schedule and taught his family members a recipe for ginseng and lotus seed soup, teaching them how to make and ingest the soup. Later, he continued exercising and eating, and he was soon on the way to recovery. He even encouraged all the patients in the cancer ward. Those who still had strength exercised with him, and those who did not began to chat with each other in the ward. He finally succeeded in fighting against his cancer, and I have only seen him when he came back to the hospital for his annual checkup.

Let me introduce here the ginseng and lotus seed soup, which can replenish energy and benefit the spleen. You can try it if you suffer from digestive tract diseases.

Ingredients: Ginseng (10 g), lotus seeds (10 pieces) , Chinese wolfberries (10 g), and rock sugar (30 g).

Cooking method: Wash the ingredients clean and soak them in clear water for 2 hours. Boil over a low heat for 1 hour.

Note: Eat only the lotus seeds, the wolfberries, and

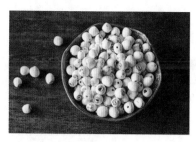

Lotus seeds.

the soup, but not the ginseng, because its energy replenishment properties are too strong.

In this recipe, we have used ginseng, because alongside replenishing energy, it has many other benefits. According to an ancient Chinese medical text, ginseng will "tone the five internal organs, pacify the spirit, calm the mind, stop heart palpitations, remove evil spirits, brighten the eyes, increase happiness, and benefit thinking and wisdom." The Chinese wolfberry nourishes the kidney and strengthens the essence. The lotus seeds not only tones the spleen, but also greatly benefits the whole digestive tract. With all these ingredients, the recipe aims to increase the patient's appetite. As long as he can eat well, his organs can maintain their operations, and he will have the strength to fight various ailments.

Irritable Bowel Syndrome

According to traditional Chinese medicine, irritable bowel syndrome consists of abdominal pain, diarrhea, and constipation. The most common symptoms include pain in the lower left part of the abdomen, diarrhea, constipation, and large amount of mucus in the feces. In feeling the lower left part of the abdomen, if you touch the spastic colon, the pain will escalate.

The most common symptom of irritable bowel syndrome is intestinal blood stasis, or intestinal spasms according to Western medicine. The patient suffering from irritable bowel syndrome has abdominal distension and pain. His feces is dry and hard, and his frequency of bowel movements increases. The excrement is thin in consistency, covered in mucus, and only comes in small amounts with each bowel movement. His tongue has a thin purple coat, which is an obvious case of blood stasis.

This ailment occurs occasionally. Some people will recover after a short bout with abdominal pain, while others may feel better only after a hospital stay. Still others regularly suffer from a sudden pain in the lower part of the abdomen. One of my patients is a ten-year-old boy. When he felt pain in the lower part of the abdomen, he reduced inflammation through blood transfusions in the hospital. As time went on, his health continued to deteriorate, and the pain increased in frequency. His aunt, who had been a friend of mine for many years, asked me to help.

I recommended a recipe called walnut and hyacinth bean paste, which the child liked to eat and which also had a healing effect. Having eaten the paste for a week, the boy no longer complained about abdominal pains. A month later, his appetite returned and he ate well.

Simple and inexpensive, this recipe has extraordinary medicinal effects. Its recipe is included here.

Ingredients: Hyacinth beans (150 g), black sesame seeds (10 g), ground walnut kernels (10 g), vegetable oil (80 g), white sugar (100 g).

Cooking method: First, prepare the hyacinth beans, peeled, and soak the beans in water. Steam the beans in a steamer for two hours. Upon taking them from the steamer, remove the water, and pound the beans into paste.

Second, bake the black sesame seeds, and grind them into powder. Heat the wok over a fire before pouring 30 g of vegetable oil into it. When the oil becomes hot, pour the paste into the work and stir-fry it until it is nearly dry. Add 50 g of white sugar into the paste and continue to stir-fry. Make sure the paste does not stick on the bottom of the wok.

Finally, add 50 g of vegetable oil, some black sesame powder, 50 g of white sugar, and the ground walnut kernels, then stir-fry the mixture for one or two minutes.

This recipe is especially good for the middle-aged and the

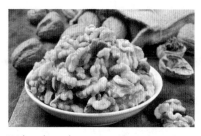

Walnut kernels.

young who suffer from irritable bowel syndrome, because it tones the spleen and stomach, benefits the intestinal tract, and increase energy and blood flow. As a further benefit, the walnut kernels and sesame will nourish the kidney and strengthen one's essence. Eating the paste regularly over a long period will help regulate the spleen and stomach, cure intestinal spasms, maintain mental tranquility, tap intellectual resources, and benefit one's study and work.

Liver and Spleen Problems

Twenty years ago, someone came to me regarding his stomach problem. I asked him whether his stomach ached more frequently an hour after eating. He thought for a while and shook his head. I asked him again, "Does it have anything to do with your emotions?" After further thought, he nodded.

Why did I ask these questions? Because in many cases, negative emotions will cause a poor appetite, which will eventually lead to stomach problems. For example, the liver governs anger, so an angry person usually does not have a good appetite. The spleen governs thinking, and if one overthinks things, he will lose his appetite. Stomachaches are often seen in two situations, spleen yang deficiency and disharmony between the liver and stomach.

According to traditional Chinese medicine, the liver corresponds to the wood element and the spleen to earth. A tree must keep absorbing nutrition from the earth to grow, which weakens the function of the earth. In other words, the liver-wood restricts the spleen-earth. Of course, under normal circumstances, the liver-wood does not restrict the spleen-earth, but it does so only when there is excessive liver-fire. When this is the case, if the patient already suffers from a spleen-stomach deficiency, he may have a stomachache and stomach distension, with pain that extends to his sides. He may even suffer from acid regurgitation, belching, bitterness in the mouth, and dysphoria. In other words, the stomachache is accompanied by the stagnation of liver energy.

I taught my patient the *xu* (see page 61) and *hu* (see page 63) breathing techniques and told him that the first technique could disperse stagnated liver energy and relieve depression, while the second could nourish the stomach and spleen. I asked him to practice the two techniques at least 6 times a day. A week later, when he came back to the hospital for a checkup, his stomachache was gone.

For those who suffer from gastritis and gastric ulcers, a gastroscopy will often reveal that their gastric mucosa is covered with either grey or purulent mucus, or is rotten or bleeding, or has ulcers. In most cases, these patients have a cold deficiency in the spleen and stomach. They feel a dull pain in the stomach, love to eat warm food, and their limbs are cold. When they press the stomach with any force, they may feel more comfortable.

When I was in the Shaolin Temple, I learned a very simple but effective method to cure stomachaches caused by a cold deficiency in the spleen and stomach. The method requires one to prepare 10 g of dry ginger and 10 pieces of pepper berries, dry them, and grind them into powder. The powder should be consumed with warm boiled water in the morning and evening. This prescription is very effective in toning the stomach and dispelling colds. When you finish drinking it, you will feel warmth in your stomach, as if a small stove were burning there.

If your stomach does not ache and you only feel cold in the stomach, you can reduce the prescription by half. Drink it every day, and you will soon get over the cold feeling in the stomach.

There is another type of stomachache caused by yin

deficiency and stomach heat. Patients suffering from this condition have a constitution with yin-deficiency, so they not only have a stomachache, but also feel dry in the mouth and suffer from heartburn. These symptoms can be relieved with lily bulb porridge, which can be made by preparing 60 g of lily bulbs and 100 g of sticky rice. These should be boiled into a porridge. Add rock sugar to taste, then eat the porridge in the morning and evening. This recipe, which nourishes the stomach and clears heat, is very effective for stomachaches caused by yin deficiency and stomach heat.

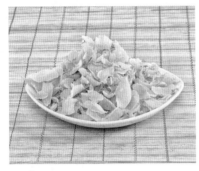

Lily bulbs.

Constipation

Constipation has many causes, which can be classified into four groups.

Pathogenic Heat Stagnated in the Lung

Constipation resulting from pathogenic heat stagnated in the lung is often caused by busyness, anxiety, and excessive internal heat. The patient also displays other symptoms, such as fever, thirst, agitation, a red tongue, and a yellow coating on the tongue.

Food Retention in the Stomach

When food is retained in the intestinal tract and blocks the smooth flow of energy in the tract, it leads to an inability to have a bowel movement. Most patients with this condition belch and have abdominal distension and acid regurgitation. They have a rotten smell in the mouth, with a red tongue and a greasy coating on the tongue.

Yin Deficiency and Low Blood Count

Patients suffering from yin deficiency and insufficient blood are often physically weak and suffer from palpitation, insomnia, and dreaminess. This is due to the yin deficiency insufficient blood, and the flaming of asthenia-fire. According to traditional Chinese medicine, blood is the mother of energy. When there is insufficient blood, one will easily feel low in energy, and the stomach and intestines will have no strength to move food down the intestinal tract, thus causing constipation.

Yang Deficiency and Coagulated Coldness

Constipation of this kind is due to insufficient function of both the spleen and the kidney. According to traditional Chinese medicine, "deficiency of yang leads to cold, which leads to coagulation." The insufficient spleen and kidney function is comparable to the absence of the sun, which results in the freezing of the land and rivers. Human beings are the same. When suffering from low function of both the spleen and the kidney, the patient will be pale-faced, with pale lips and tongue, and a white coating on the tongue. They eat less and are in low spirits.

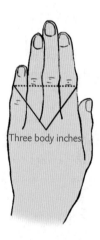

Three body inches

Two acupuncture points can effectively help relax the bowels. They are located three body inches away from the navel, with one on the right and the other on the left. (As the figure on the left shows, the length of the broken line between the index finger and the little finger is three body inches.) If the constipation is not serious, rub each of the points for three minutes, and it will result in easier bowel movements. If this does not help, you should consult a doctor for appropriate treatment.

Diarrhea

Mr. Liu consulted me about his illness. When we chatted, his eyes turned red. At age 37, he should have been working hard for a better life. However, he had lost several jobs and was now staying at home, unemployed. He said, "This is all due to diarrhea. I got my driver's license at 22 and drove a truck, earning quite a lot of money. Life was good until 5 years ago, when I got chronic uncontrollable diarrhea. On one occasion, I even failed to control my bowels when I was driving. From that time on, I have not had a chance to drive. Later, I worked in a restaurant and conducted some small business, but the diarrhea ruined that opportunity as well. Now I stay at home like a good-for-nothing, supported by my wife."

He was emaciated and pale-faced, with drooping eyelids and bent back. His palm was much colder than mine. His tongue was swollen, and the coating on his tongue was thin and white. Obviously, his chronic diarrhea was caused by low function of both the spleen and the kidney. According to traditional Chinese medicine, the kidney governs containment and the spleen manages transportation and transformation. The low function of both spleen and kidney causes abnormal transportation and transformation and the weakening of containment, which ultimately results in diarrhea.

I asked this patient to return home and do the following exercises. First, practice the standing exercise (see page 87) 20 to 30 minutes a day to replenish energy and improve the constitution. Second, practice the *chui* breathing technique (see page 66) at least 6 times a day. Third, rub the stomach, the waist, and the Yongquan point anti-clockwise 36 times each. The second and third exercises would help tone yang in the kidney. Last, I instructed him to rub the Tianshu points from outside in 36 times. The Tianshu points, which correspond to the large intestine, are the best means to cure diarrhea. They are located two body inches away from the navel, one on the right and the other on the left.

Half a month later, Mr. Liu had normal bowel movements once to twice a day.

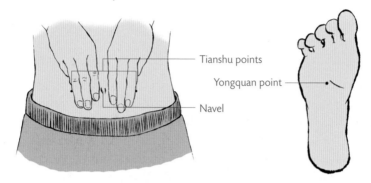

Tianshu points

Yongquan point

Navel

Another type of diarrhea is caused by weakness of the spleen and stomach. The weakness of the spleen and stomach cause the food that enters the stomach to be discharged from the intestinal tract without sufficient digestion and absorption. To cure this ailment, one can use a simple but effective Zen prescription from the Shaolin Temple.

Prepare an appropriate amount of hazelnut kernels, roasting them in a wok, until yellow. Grind the kernel into fine powder and put the powder into a bottle. Boil a bowl of water with two red dates in it to make a half bowl of soup. Take a spoonful of the powder from the bottle for each serving and eat it with the soup.

Hazelnut kernels can tone the spleen and stomach and increase physical strength. Red date soup is good for enhancing the efficacy of the medicine, because the red date nourishes the spleen and stomach and aids the absorption of the medicine.

2. Orthopedic Disorders

If we compare the human body to a machine, the legs, bones, and joints are the engine. If the engine does not work well, the machine will naturally age and fail to operate properly.

A farmer once came to me, telling me that he had contracted a strange disease, growing colder and colder from the waist to the feet. At night, even when he covered himself with two quilts, he could not get warm. He had to use a hot water bottle to warm himself up, even in autumn.

He also told me that he had been to many hospitals and undergone many tests, including kidney function test and CT scans of the abdomen, which cost him a lot of money, but still failed to uncover the cause of the ailment.

After examining his tests carefully, I found that his internal organs were all fine, the flexibility of his blood vessels was extremely good, and he did not have high blood pressure, hyperlipidemia, or hyperglycemia. Then I said to him, "There's no problem with your health, but as you age, your legs age first. The energy in your lower limbs does not flow smoothly, and this results in energy stagnation and blood stasis. For this reason, little energy can reach the legs, and that leads you to feel cold down from the waist. But generally, there's nothing wrong with your health."

In fact, apart from the disharmony between energy and blood in his lower limbs, the farmer's ailment had a great deal to do with the decrease of his kidney function. This is normal, because, as a man of over 50, he could not escape the laws of nature. However, we can slow the aging of our internal organs with various methods, which will in turn slow the aging in our limbs.

Leg and Foot Weakness

Many people are surprised when I tell them my age, saying that I look at least 20 years younger. My secret is to maintain the health of my legs and feet, because, as an old Chinese saying goes, the tree withers at its roots first, and as we age, our legs weaken first. Our legs have been at work from the moment we were born to the time we die. As we grow older, they will naturally be in poor condition if we do not protect them.

With the development of science and technology, we have more means of transportation. The chances for us to use our legs are decreasing. As a result, our legs gradually become weaker. That's why we find people whose legs ache severely even when they walk a short distance, not to mention climbing mountains.

Many people feel that the *qigong* of the Shaolin Temple is very powerful. This is because the warrior-monks emphasized the training of their legs. As long as our legs are solid and strong, we look spirited and can walk with great vigor. Therefore, in order to enjoy good health, we must have healthy legs.

Most importantly, we should keep our legs warm. To do so, we can regularly soak our feet in warm water. In addition, instead of staying indoors, we should exercise more and spend time in the sun. We can walk in sunny weather, which helps cultivate our body and soul, and also makes our legs strong.

To conclude, if we take good care of our legs, we will look much younger.

Lumbar Disc Herniation

When one laughs hard, his body will uncontrollably rock forwards and backwards. In fact, as simple as it is, this "rocking"

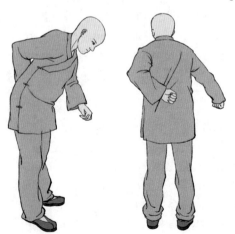

movement is effective in curing lumbar disc herniation.

The "rocking" technique includes standing with your body fully relaxed and your fists clenched. Press your thumbs against your index and middle fingers. Bend forward to about 30 degrees while hitting the elixir field with your left hand and the right side of the small of the back with your right hand. Then, arch your body backwards slowly, keeping your legs straight, and shake your arms as you hit the elixir field with your right land and the left side of the small of the back with your left hand. (The sides of the small of the back are the spot your hands touch when you shake your hands naturally back and forth.) In addition, make sure that you do not hit both hands against the body at the same time, but alternately.

This exercise makes you feel very comfortable. You must persevere, but you don't need to overdo it. One or two hundred times a day is enough.

Body Aches

Many people do not exercise. They ache all over when they play volleyball or join in a group exercise on rare occasions, and they do not recover for many days. In addition, there are many middle-aged and elderly people who suffer from body aches or random pains (also known as scurrying pain). For these people, the serpentine technique might be effective.

The serpentine technique is very simple, requiring the practitioner to move forward like a snake. It involves standing with the body fully relaxed, your feet and legs together, and your hands against the seams of your pants. Move your head forward and shrug your shoulders in unison, creating an S-shape with your body. Repeat this movement, as if moving like a snake.

After you finish the exercise, you will feel comfortable all over, as if each of the joints were oiled. Practicing this movement regularly will make you feel that your body aches are relieved, while will allow you to have a good night of sleep.

Cervical Spondylosis

In the past, cervical spondylosis was often found in people above 40. Today, it is now common in younger people as well. Some patients with cervical spondylosis may feel pain, numbness, or a lack of strength in one shoulder and arm, and their necks may not be able to move easily. Others may feel dizzy or even sick when they stand or move their heads. These restrictions affect their lives and work quite severely. In fact, most middle-aged patients who get this disease, a degenerative ailment, find that it is the result of long-time strain. In young patients, it is often acute, but if they persevere, they can fully recover.

When you feel discomfort in the cervical vertebra, there are several methods that may bring some relief.

Relaxing the Neck Muscles
The patient should sit on a chair. While the doctor stands behind him and rubs his neck and shoulders for about 3 minutes, massaging each point 5 to 6 times. This relaxes the muscle group in the neck.

Restituting the Neck Joints
The patient bends his head forward to about 30 degrees. The doctor presses the spinous process on the patient's 7th cervical vertebra with his right thumb, supporting the patient's lower jaw with his left elbow as he pulls the jaw upwards, then slowly turns the patient's head to the side. Repeat this 5 to 6 times.

Pulling the Neck
The patient lies on the bed, shoulders propped up with a pillow. The doctor stands beside the bed, right hand holding the pillow and left hand holding the patient's upper jaw. The patient's head is raised slowly from the pillow until it forms a 45 degree angle with the bed. The traction is held for 2 minutes. Finally, the patient should gently move the head right and left, then back and forth, making each movement three times.

Rubbing the Cervical Vertebra with Warm Palms
The doctor rubs his palms until they grow warm, then massages both sides of the patient's neck with warm palms, 6 times on each side. Finally, he rubs directly on both sides of the patient's

cervical vertebra until his hands grow warm.

The patient should be treated with this method every night for at least one week.

Back and Leg Soreness

When we get old, we will inevitably have trouble with our muscles and bones, including stiffness and aches at the waist, an inability to sit for long periods, and heaviness at the waist when rising in the morning. The symptoms will be somewhat relieved after exercise, but they will become serious with excessive work. In the most serious cases, the patient cannot even bend down.

Ms. Niu came to me with a lower back ache. When I inquired her about the causes, she answered, "When I was 32, we were building our own house. I fell from a scaffold as tall as a man and hurt my waist. From that time on, I have suffered a dull pain in the lower back. Before, I could still do light work, but in the past two years, my lower back has not only ached, but has also become stiff and hard. Now, I can't sit up in the morning, and getting out of bed is a torture."

I asked her to lie on her stomach on the bed and massaged her Jiaji points (the Jiaji point is located at 0.5 body inches away from both sides of the spine between the first thoracic vertebra and the fifth lumbar vertebra, with 34 points altogether, 17 on each side) with the end of my right palm up from the

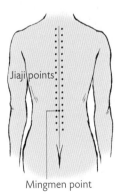

Jiaji points

Mingmen point

tailbone. I rubbed 6 times in total, then massaged the lower back horizontally 6 times. Finally, I put one hand onto the other and pressed the Mingmen point 100 times.

She sat up from the bed, stood on the ground, and stretched her lower back, feeling much better. I told her to ask her husband to massage her back this way every morning and evening.

Rubbing the Jiaji points can dredge the yang channel and nourish the internal organs. Massaging the lower back horizontally can condition the psoas muscles, while pressing the Mingmen point can strengthen the kidney and bones.

Acute Lumbar Muscle Sprain

When the monks in the Shaolin Temple practice martial arts, they inevitably get injured. For example, acute lumbar sprain is very common among them. When I was young, I saw many monks in the temple who suffered a lumbar muscle sprain, but none of them had lain in bed for several days to recover. This was because they had a secret formula that involved relaxing the muscles through the "rolling" method.

In the rolling method, the doctor clenches his fist gently and uses the back of his hand and the protruding digital joints to keep rolling back and forth on the painful point, moving slowly while rolling. He repeats the action along the musculus sacrospinalis fiber (located close to the hunch on both sides of the spine) beside the injured point 6 times. He then putting the palm on the injured place and raises the leg on the side of the injury 3 times. Next, he plucks at the injured point with his right hand to stimulate the circulation of blood and cause the muscles and joints to relax, rubbing the musculus sacrospinalis on the side of the injury with his right palm until his hand gets warm. Finally, he pats the spine from top to bottom to dredge the channels all over the patient's body.

Generally, after the above treatment is done, many patients will have less pain or no pain at all. They will usually go home on their own. The patient should refrain from twisting his lower back or arching the backs backwards for at least a week. He should also stop doing intense work.

Strain of Lumbar Muscles

Mr. Zhou and his wife ran a small restaurant. He was the chef while his wife worked as the waitress. As time went by, his lower back began to ache intermittently. A medical check found that he had strained his lumbar muscles.

Lumbar strains can be treated with massage. The steps for this massage are listed here.

❶ Rub the bladder meridian on both sides of the lower back (see page 142) 15 times each, from top to bottom with the end of a palm, then rub the lumbosacral portion horizontally 15 times.

❷ Pat each of the muscle groups on the lower back 15 times with a hollow fist.

❸ Massage the Weizhong points and the Chengshan points. The Weizhong points, which are very easy to find, are located at the depressions in the center of the hamstrings of the legs. Press the thumb against the Weizhong point and then loose it, which makes the patient feel very comfortable. You can press the two points with both thumbs 100 times. The Weizhong point is well-known for relieving pain, and therefore, if you suffer from prosopalgia, backache, and knee aches, you can try this method.

The Chengshan point is close to the Weizhong point. When you stretch your lower leg, you will find a protruding part on the back of the calf. This is the Chengshan point. There is one on the back of each of the lower legs. Press the Chengshan points in the same manner you press the Weizhong points, 100 times each. Massaging the Chengshan points can also relieve lower back and leg pain.

If you suffer from lumbar muscles strain that has extended to your thighs, you can press the Huantiao point. This point is not hard to find, either. When you tense your buttocks, you will find a depression on each buttock, and that is the Huantiao point. Massaging this point can treat diseases below the thighs. The patient can ask his family member to press each of the points 100 times with the elbow.

What Mr. Zhou had was acute strain of lumbar muscles. Since he was young and had just sustained the injury, it was easy

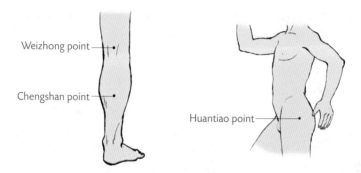

Weizhong point

Chengshan point

Huantiao point

to cure. However, for those with long-term strains of the lumbar muscles, along with the above methods, they can also regularly eat rice porridge with chestnuts. The method of cooking this porridge is presented here.

Prepare 100 g of chestnuts, shells removed, and 50 g of rice, washed clean. Put these into a wok and boil them in water. Add white sugar to taste.

The main ingredient is the chestnut, which benefits the spleen, stomach, and kidney meridians and can nourish the spleen and stomach, reinforce the kidney, activate blood, and strengthen tendons and bones. However, eating too much of it can cause stagnation of the circulation of vital energy and excessive internal heat. Therefore, I do not recommend it be consumed directly, but only as part of the porridge.

To conclude, strain of the lumbar muscles is caused by excessive fatigue. Therefore, the patient needs to be taken good care of the injury at home, and the best care his family members can give is to aid in massages and food therapy.

3. Cardio-Cerebral Diseases

When our brains suffer from tension or high pressure over a prolonged period, our ability to conduct mental activities will wane. For example, aside from bodily discomforts, we will also be prone to irritation and mental fatigue, and we will suffer from sleep disorders, absent-mindedness, forgetfulness, headaches, and other bodily discomforts. Some patients may have fanciful thoughts and find it difficult to fall asleep. Their minds will go off into wild flights of fancy.

Today, many people are troubled with neurasthenia. They are busy with their work, seldom exercise, and love socializing and drinking alcohol. Consequently, they get high blood pressure and hyperlipidemia.

Some entrepreneurs often come to me for their diseases. They usually say, "My brain doesn't work anymore. I keep forgetting things. I even forget what others just said to me." This is a typical example of neurasthenia caused by overwork and an excessive exertion of brain power.

Once I had a friend who engaged in futures trading and was very wealthy. He recommended a patient to me, his office director. When the patient came to me, he told me that futures trading was not good now, that he was under great pressure, and that he must read extensively every day just to keep up with trends. When I asked what seemed to be his trouble, he answered, "I'm forgetful and easily feel dizzy. I feel bored reading report forms and business proposals. My ears ring, I don't sleep well, and I dream a lot. I've been like this for more than half a year."

His symptoms had to do with liver fire ascending that was burning heart yin and he needed to clear away the liver fire and heat and promote diuresis.

There are also people who suffer from insomnia and dreaminess, palpitations and restlessness, and dizziness and forgetfulness, due to low functioning heart and spleen and deficiency of energy and blood count. They also show other symptoms of poor spleen function, such as abdominal distension, poor appetite, pallor, and emancipation.

Others suffer from neurasthenia because of a heart-kidney imbalance. Since the heart governs fire and the kidney governs water, when there is an imbalance between the heart and kidney, the heart fire cannot descend to warm the kidney water, which in turn cannot ascend to nourish the heart fire. The patient will then experience palpitations, restlessness, anxiety, and insomnia. He may also have other kidney-related symptoms, such as hair loss, forgetfulness, soreness and weakness of the lower back and knees, night sweats, and spermatorrhea.

In fact, the more we use our brains, the more flexible they become. However, we must also give them enough rest to maintain healthy operation.

Myocardial Ischemia

When I was young, a man visited my grandpa to treat his illness. He said that he felt tightness in the chest and a lack of strength all day long, which, in modern terms, is myocardial ischemia.

He told my grandpa that he did not have too much money. My grandfather asked him whether he could afford to eat an egg every day, and he said he could. Then, my grandpa said, "Go and

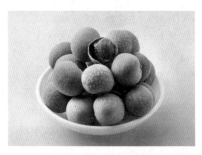

Longans.

buy some longans. Boil a pot of water every morning, pour it into a bowl, and whip an egg into the water. Cover the bowl with a lid for 5 minutes, and then put into it 7 longans. Eat this for 100 days, and you'll recover fully."

Following this inexpensive prescription, the man eventually recovered.

Eggs are nutritious, and longans benefit the heart and spleen, nourish the blood, and soothe the nerves. They can be used for elderly people who suffer from low energy and low blood count, shortness of breath, and fatigue, and for women confined to bed because they suffer from excessive hemorrhaging.

This method is one I used frequently when I later became a doctor, and it proved effective every time. I often share it with middle-aged and elderly friends who suffer from myocardial ischemia and palpitations. They generally feel more vigorous and experience a complete change if they persevere with this method for about 100 days.

Alzheimer's Disease

At the gate of the Temple, there is a vigorous elderly woman who sells joss sticks and candles. Visitors who buy from her are often astonished at her mental power. She can figure out more quickly than a calculator how much a buyer should pay, needing just seconds, even when the customer buys a big pile of joss sticks and candles. This woman is my mother, aged 91.

However, 20 years ago, my mother was not like this. Her brain did not work well, and she was forgetful. Her fast thinking now is the result of a finger exercise I taught her.

The method involves stretching your arms, with one of them at the 4 o'clock position and the other at the 8 o'clock position. Raise your arms slightly, clench your fists, with your thumbs pressing against the other four fingers and your palms facing backwards. Then, stretch your fingers out one by one from the little finger, to the ring finger, to the middle finger, to the index finger, and finally to the thumb. Turn the palms forward simultaneously, like two flowers gradually blooming. When all the fingers are stretched and the palms face forward, withdraw your fingers one by one from the little fingers and turn your palms backwards at the same time. Don't move too fast when you first learn the method, or the result will be cut in half. Practice this method 150 times every morning.

Why is this method an effective exercise for the brain? Because, according to traditional Chinese medicine, the nerves in the fingertips are linked with the heart, which governs the spirit and commands the whole body. Exercising the fingers,

then, can make the heart blood vigorous and cause the mind
to react more quickly. According to discoveries in modern
physiological research, each part of the human body, such as the
hand and feet, has a reflex zone in the brain. It is the reflex zone
that enables the brain to command all the body parts. Since the
hands are the most flexible, their reflex zone in the brain is the
largest, making up one third of the area of all reflex zones. With
the method I teach, one third of the reflex zones in the brain get
exercise, and you will certainly become more quick-witted.

Excessive Internal Heat

In the modern society, people work in a fast paced environment
and do things at a hectic pace. As a result, they are prone to
excessive internal heat.

A very simple method to lower internal heat is to eat more
celery. When one suffers from excessive internal heat, he will
have physical problems such as feverish palms and soles, oral
ulcers, constipation, and mental problems such as agitation and
irritability.

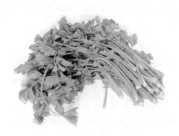

Celery.

Celery can clear away
heat, calm the liver, and
moisten the intestines.
According to traditional
Chinese medicine, the liver
stores blood and governs
anger, and it can, therefore,
pacify the liver fire and make
one calm down. Since celery
also moistens the intestines and aids bowel movements, it can
also serve as the cleanser of the intestines, which, once clean,
can make the fire and heat disappear by themselves, naturally
relieving related symptoms.

I recommend patients buy celery every day, wash it, and cut
it into small sections. It should then be warmed in boiled water

for 1 minute. After adding condiments, it can be eaten.

Once I had a student whose lips often became dry due to excessive internal heat. He often drank three to four cups of water in the morning when he first became my patient. Even so, his urine was still very yellow and his feces very dry. I told him, "You can't drink that much water, because your kidneys' ability to metabolize water is limited. Too much water will add a burden to the kidneys, which will cause kidney problems in the long run." I recommended he eat celery.

After eating celery for a month, he told me, "Master, my lupus erythematosus is gone."

I was surprised at his words, but then understood. Lupus erythematosus has a great deal to do with the flourishing of an internal heat toxin. After he ate celery for a prolonged period, the heat toxin was removed, and so was the lupus erythematosus.

Cardiac Infarction

Cardiac infarction means that the heart and blood vessels are blocked. If the small vessel is blocked, the patient will feel chest pains, palpitation, and similar discomforts. If the main artery is blocked, his life will be endangered.

Generally, heart disease patients will usually prepare medicine at home, just in case the disease breaks out. However, many patients may not have time to get to the medicine if they have a sudden heart attack. Even when the medicine is right before them, they may lack the strength to grab it. In addition, many middle-aged and young people who are not diagnosed with heart diseases, and therefore prepare no medicine at home, may similarly suffer sudden cardiac infarction.

What can we do in these circumstances? Very simple. If you get a sudden heart attack, immediately take a deep breath and then hold it for at least a dozen seconds. Many people have come around this way.

Of course, whatever happens, if you have medicine at hand,

take it while you hold your breath. At the very least, you should try to make noise by beating the table or something similar to alert your family members, who will then call for help.

Angina Pectoris

Angina pectoris can cause paroxysmal chest pain, usually behind the breast bone. Although it does not last long, the patient feels as if a huge stone were placed on his chest, and some may even experience crushing pain, like a knife being twisted in the hearts. Others may feel that they are on the verge of death.

Judging from traditional Chinese medicine, there are four types of angina pectoris.

Heart Energy Deficiency

Patients suffering from deficient heart energy generally feel insipid and dispirited. They do not like talking, suffer from tightness in the chest and shortness of breath, and have a light-colored tongue with a white coating. They can practice the *he* and *chui* breathing techniques (mainly inhaling) (see pages 62 and 66) in the morning and evening 6 times each day and take a happy walk (with long inhalations and short exhalations) (see page 90) twice a day, each lasting 30–40 minutes. The *he* breathing technique nourishes the heart, and the *chui* breathing technique nourishes the kidney. Used together, they can replenish heart energy, reinforce nephrons, and increase yang energy.

Heart Yin Deficiency

Patients suffering from heart yin deficiency are mostly troubled by dysphoria, insomnia, feverish palms and soles, sweating, excessive water intake, and dry feces. They can practice the *he* breathing technique (short inhalations and long exhalations) to clear heart fire. However, since most patients with this condition are physically weak, they also need to reinforce their nephrons with the *chui* breathing technique (long inhalations and short exhalations). The healing effect will be intensified if they can take a happy walk (short inhalations and long exhalations) twice a day, each lasting 30–40 minutes.

Heart Blood Stasis

When attacked by angina pectoris, some patients feel severe pain at a fixed place, the Danzhong point, which is located at the central point between the nipples. When suffering from this condition, the tongue is dark purple with ecchymoses on it. This type of angina pectoris is mainly caused by heart blood stasis.

Heart blood stasis endangers the patient's life, because it can easily result in blood vessel blockage and cause cardiac infarction. The painful point is the precise spot where the blood stasis is located. The patient can rub with force on the Danzhong point with the thenar eminence every morning and evening, 100 times each. Meanwhile, he can practice the *he* breathing technique 6 times each morning and evening and take a slow happy walk (mainly long inhalation, short exhalations, and slow steps) twice a day, based on his physical condition, each lasting 30–40 minutes.

Phlegm Blocking the Heart Vessels

Some angina pectoris patients may suffer from nausea and abdominal distension, tightness in the chest, and shortness of breath. If their tongues are light-colored with a white and greasy coat, their disease is probably caused by phlegm blocking the heart vessels. Such patients should practice the *he* and *hu* (see page 63) breathing techniques, mainly exhalations. They should also take a happy walk (mainly long exhalations) twice a day, each lasting 30–40 minutes.

In fact, all types of angina pectoris are related to cardiovascular blockages. When the heart and blood vessels are blocked, the patient feels pain. Therefore, we need to take precautions when we are diagnosed with myocardial ischemia. It can also be treated with the food therapy laid out below.

Prepare the same amount of purslane and Chinese leeks,

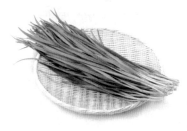

Chinese leeks.

washing them separately, then dry them in the shade for two hours and cut them into small pieces. Fry several eggs to taste. Cut the eggs into tiny shreds, mix it with the vegetables, and add condiments. Prepared steamed buns with this filling and eat them regularly.

The purslane in this recipe cools the blood and dissipates blood stasis, while the Chinese leek warms and nourishes the kidneys. Eating these ingredients over a prolonged period prevents heart diseases and promotes longevity.

High Blood Pressure

Cerebral vessel raptures and myocardial infarctions, which cause great harm to the human body, are chiefly brought about by high blood pressure. The blood vessels are like a dam, and the blood is like the river water. When the blood pressure increases, the river begins to overflow, beating against the vascular walls without stopping. As time passes, the vascular walls will become less flexible and the arteries will gradually harden. If we allow the blood pressure to continue to rise, sooner or later, the cerebral vessel will break, causing cerebral hemorrhaging. If the cerebral vessel is blocked, we will have cerebral infarction. The same is true of the heart and blood vessels. It is important to take action to control the blood pressure as early as possible.

Most patients I encountered in the hospital had high blood pressure caused by excessive liver yang. What on earth is excessive liver yang? Let me explain with an analogy. The cold weather in northern China requires heating in winter. As long as the fire is hot, the water that flows through the pipes will remain hot. Similarly, the liver fire in the body of the patient who suffers from excessive liver yang provides heat to the blood in the vessels that keeps impacting the heart and brain. Therefore, these patients usually suffer from headaches, insomnia, agitation, and a bitter taste in the mouth. They also have flushed faces, and the tip of their tongues are red.

It is highly recommended that these patients practice the *xu* breathing technique (see page 61), especially when their blood pressure rises. They should also check their blood pressure daily and take a happy walk (see page 90) in the morning and evening, for 30–40 minutes each time.

For some, their high blood pressure has to do with the deficiency of liver yin and kidney yin. They often experience headaches, dizziness, ringing in the ears, soreness and weakness of the lower back and knees, palpitations, irritability, insomnia, and forgetfulness, and their tongues are red and dry. At this point, you might have felt a little confused. Aren't these symptoms the same as high blood pressure caused by excess of the liver yang?

No, they are not the same. Symptoms such as headaches, insomnia, palpitations, and irritability are linked with the liver, which stores blood and governs anger. However, the kidneys, which govern the bones, which in turn generate marrow, opens at the ears. Therefore, dizziness, ringing in the ear, soreness and weakness of the lower back and knees, and forgetfulness relate to the kidney. If a patient has all these symptoms at the same time, it is certain that his high blood pressure is caused by a deficiency of liver yin and kidney yin. He should practice both the *xu* breathing technique and the *chui* breathing technique (see page 66), and he should also take a happy walk every morning and evening for 30–40 minutes each time.

Whichever type of high blood pressure you might suffer from, you can treat it with the celery porridge.

To cook celery porridge, prepare 100 g of celery, keeping its roots and leaves. Wash the celery and cut it into tiny shreds. Boil 100 g of rice in water in a wok and put the celery shreds into the wok to boil after the porridge is cooked. Eat the porridge every morning and evening. It will invigorate the stomach, have a diuretic effect, tranquilize the mind, and reduce blood pressure.

In addition, tea therapy can also help lower blood pressures. Prepare 5 g of saffron and 10 g of red dates and hawthorn berries each. Wash these ingredients clean, put them in water, and drink the water.

Both saffron and hawthorn berry can reduce blood pressure. They also help activate blood, remove stasis, burn fat, and aid in weight loss. Those who suffer from high blood pressure can drink a cup of this tea every day. They can also bring this tea with them when they work or travel.

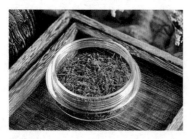

Saffron.

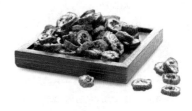

Hawthorn berries.

4. Respiratory System

Shaolin masters often drink Zen tea, when means that when the tea is ready, they first take a deep breath of the hot rising steam and appreciate the tea fragrance with eyes closed before finally taking a sip of the tea. As time goes by, I have also formed this habit, even when I am drinking a cup of water.

One winter, the weather was extremely dry. Several doctors and nurses in my department got colds and were troubled with sore throats and fever. When we were chatting, one doctor said casually, "It's very dry this winter. Even my nostrils feel dry."

At that time, I was holding a cup of water in my hands. Sniffing it, I took a sip. It was true that winter was very dry, but I did not feel it at all. In addition, I seldom got colds. Later, I gradually discovered that the reason lay in the way I drank water.

Every day, when my eyes were tired from writing prescriptions, I put my eyes over the cup and let the hot steam circle around them. Nourished by the steam, my eyes brightened.

Every time I felt dry in the nostrils during dry weather, I sniffed the steam from the boiled water I was about to drink, then exhaled it through the mouth. Repeating this several times, my nose was moistened.

Every time I had talked myself hoarse and dry, I took a deep breath over my cup, drawing in the hot steam, then exhaled it through my nose. Doing this several times, I felt that the soreness in my throat had been greatly relieved. It was faster and more effective than taking a throat lozenge.

When a woman feels dry, her face will lack luster or even desquamate, and as time passes, she may develop wrinkles earlier than expected. Applying facial masks or toners can be time-consuming or even hurt the facial skin. In this case, she can try leaning over a bowl of boiled water and soak her face in the hot steam.

I taught this method to my daughter. When she was in junior and senior middle schools, the tight learning schedule led most of her classmates to start wearing glasses, but my daughter's eyesight remained good, and she seldom caught colds.

Colds

The warrior-monks in the Shaolin Temple practice martial arts daily and are generally very strong. However, they occasionally also catch colds. When this is the case, the master will take a pinch of white pepper powder, cut an onion into small sections, and boil these ingredients in water with several slices of ginger. He will then take these ingredients out and boil some noodles in the soup, along with some condiments. After eating the noodles with the soup, the patient will cover his head with the quilt and have a good sleep. As he perspires, the cold will be relieved.

This method is effective for slight colds. There are several types of colds.

The Wind-Cold Type of Common Cold
The wind-cold type of common cold is basically the same as a common cold caused by cold weather. The symptoms include a runny nose, cough, and sneezing. The patient can try the above white pepper powder noodles to treat this type of cold.

The Wind-Heat Type of Common Cold
The symptoms include fever, headaches, yellow nasal mucus, dry mouth, swollen and sore throat, yellow phlegm, yellow tongue coating, and similar symptoms. The patient can treat this with the tea therapy described below.

Prepare 10 g of honeysuckle and chrysanthemum each, 30 g of folia pleioblasti, 5 g of mulberry leaves, and 2 g of mint. These are ingredients for medicine or tea that can clear away heat, relieve external symptoms, and disperse wind. They are available in TCM pharmacies. Put these ingredients into a teapot and soak them in boiled water for 2 minutes before drinking. The effect will be better if you use a thermos teapot.

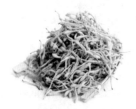
Honeysuckle.

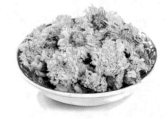
Chrysanthemum.

The Exterior Cold and Interior Heat Type of Cold
The symptoms of this sort of cold consist either headaches, body

aches, chills, and nasal obstructions caused by external cold, or of fever, thirst, sore throat, yellow phlegm, yellow urine, and dry feces caused by internal heat. This sort of cold can be treated with the soup described here.

Prepare 200 g of white radish, wash it clean, and cut it into small pieces. Boil the radish pieces together with 5 olives in plain water, making soup. Eat a small bowl of the soup three times a day. This recipe can clear away heat and remove toxicity. It is also effective in preventing flu.

Acute Coughs

After recovering from a cold, some people may continue to suffer from a dry cough without phlegm. They even cough so severely they wake up at night. When they do have phlegm, they find it hard to get rid of it, which makes them feel miserable.

In traditional Chinese medicine, this is known as an irritating dry cough, which is characterized by a dry cough without phlegm or slight but thick phlegm that cannot be totally eliminated. It usually occurs when the patient seems to have recovered from a cold. Since the focus of a cold infection is mostly in the nose and throat, when the symptoms there improve, the cold seems to be cured. But this is far from true. The focus of the infection simply moves down the respiratory system to the bronchial tube, causing acute bronchitis, as it is called in Western medicine.

In fact, an irritating dry cough is nothing serious, according to traditional Chinese medicine. There is no need for the patient to take antibiotics. These patients require only a sesame and rock sugar drink.

Put 15 g of raw sesame and 10 g of rock sugar into boiled water and drink it three times a day, half an hour before each meals. The cough will be relieved within two or three days.

Since an irritating dry cough is caused by two factors, irritation and cough, we should first nourish the yin and generate body fluid, then stop the cough. In this recipe, the sesame benefits the lung, kidney, and spleen, prevents cough, and increases the immunity of the body. The rock sugar, on the other hand, moistens the lung, stops the cough, and clears away phlegm.

In addition, the patient can also adopt the *xi* breathing technique (mainly through exhalation) to clear away the lung heat, and the *chui* breathing technique (mainly through inhalation) (see pages 66 and 67) to replenish the kidney energy and increase immunity.

Chronic Bronchitis

When a cold is not thoroughly treated, it will turn into an acute cough, which, in turn, will result in a chronic cough if not completely cured. Patients with chronic coughs generally suffer from chronic bronchitis. They often cough and spit, and they are more likely to do so in winter or when the weather suddenly turns cold. The symptoms will be relieved or simply vanish when it turns warm.

If you listen with a stethoscope to the upper and lower parts, especially the lower part, of the lung of a chronic bronchitis patient, you will hear dry or moist sounds, an abnormal respiratory sound characterized by small crackles. They are either coarse or fine-grained, and they are heard in different parts of the lung. An X-ray will find an increase of pulmonary shadows and lung markings.

Chronic bronchitis recurs easily and affects the emotional state of the patient. According to traditional Chinese medicine, the lung governs sadness, so the patient may easily feel depressed.

Yang Tan (1120–1185), a famous doctor of traditional Chinese medicine in the Song dynasty (960–1279), created a fine prescription for curing chronic bronchitis, recording it in a medical book he wrote. I have reproduced it here.

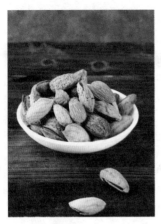

Sweet almonds.

Ingredients: Sweet almonds (250 g), walnut kernels (500 g), and honey (500 g).

Cooking method: First, bake the sweet almonds until golden, but do not overbake them. Boil some water with these sweet almonds in a wok for one hour, then pound the walnut kernels into pieces and put them into the wok. Over a low flame, boil and add honey when the water is nearly dried up. Finally, stir contents well, boil again, then switch off the fire. Eat this in the morning and evening, 3 g each time.

This prescription is simple but effective. The sweet almonds have two major functions, diffusing the inhibited lung energy and relieving cough, which is a temporary solution, and warming and toning the lungs, which is a permanent cure. The walnut kernels also have two functions, relieving the cough and preventing asthma (long term coughs may cause asthma), and toning the kidneys and strengthening resistance. According to traditional Chinese medicine, "Since long term coughs affects the kidneys, a cough will not be cured unless the kidneys are cured." This prescription not only moistens the lungs and relieves the cough, but also reinforces and tones the body.

Pulmonary Emphysema

When I was young, I stayed in the Shaolin Temple. There I often saw the nearby villagers who came to the temple for their diseases. Among them were some old patients with pulmonary emphysema who breathed with great difficulty, coughed a lot, and had excessive phlegm. Seeing this, the Zen doctor in the temple would pluck a section from the pumpkin vine in the field and insert it into a bottle. After one night, the juice from the vine would flow into the bottle. The next morning, the master would ask the patient to drink the juice with water and instruct him to practice the *xi*, *hu*, and *chui* breathing techniques (see pages 63, 66 and 67), supplemented with a happy walk (see page 90). Gradually, the patients' symptoms were greatly relieved.

The pulmonary emphysema many elderly people suffer relates to phlegm generated by poor spleen function. Cough and phlegm also occur when the lung yin is deficient or the lung has a depressive fire. Pumpkin vine juice, which is bitter and slightly cold, can nourish the spleen, moisten the lungs, and harmonize the stomach. In this way, it restrains pulmonary emphysema.

The problem is that the pumpkin vine is not available all year round. As a substitute, I recommend an eight-treasure porridge, which the patient can have regardless of season.

Ingredients: Almonds (6 g), peach seeds (6 g), walnut kernels (10 g), Gorgon fruit (20 g), coix seeds (20 g), lily bulbs (20 g), peanut kernels (30 g), and gingko nuts (20 g) (with shells removed).

Cooking method: Boil these ingredients in water for 20 minutes, then add 100 g of rice and cook into a porridge.

Finish the porridge in two portions within a day. For patients with a larger appetite, the porridge can be eaten in one serving. This recipe tones the kidneys, strengthens the spleen, diffuses inhibited lung energy, and relieves coughs.

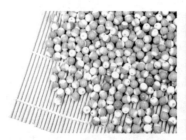

Gorgon fruit.

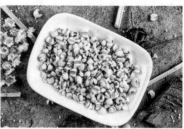

Coix seeds.

Coughs

More than 20 years ago when I was working in a hospital, an elderly man came for a consultation. He was emaciated, and his eyes were lifeless. As soon as he saw me, he said, "Doctor, I'm coughing up blood. Am I going to die?"

When I asked him about the causes, his sons and daughters told me that he had had a chronic cough for more than a dozen years, but he had begun to cough blood only recently. Having brought him to various doctors who had failed to cure him, they brought him to me.

I asked him to do an X-ray and a bronchoscopy. The X-ray showed no shadows, eliminating the possibility of lung cancer. The bronchoscopy indicated that his bronchial wall was congested, thickened, and enlarged, and some parts were even bleeding.

Now it was clear that the old man had bronchiectasis, the typical symptoms of which were cough, asthma, excessive phlegm, and hemoptysis.

I gave him a careful examination. His phlegm was yellow and sticky, and it had blood in it. In addition, he had a dry mouth, flushed tongue, and his tongue had a yellow coat. This was obviously caused by lung heat that injured the pulmonary collaterals.

"What you have is not cancer, but bronchiectasis. You will recover if you keep exercising," I told the elderly man.

Then I demonstrated to him how to do the exercise. First, forcefully massage the thenar eminence in the direction of the forearm, then rub the Chize point from inside (the little finger side) to the outside (the thumb side). The Chize point is very easy to find (see next page). Raise your arm and you can find a thick tendon in the center of the inner side of the arm. The point is located at the outer side of the tendon.

Rubbing these two points would clear the heat in the lungs. After this, I instructed him to slowly rub the Taixi point in a

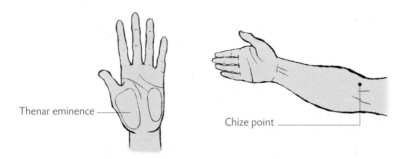

Thenar eminence

Chize point

clockwise movement. The Taixi point is located in the depression
in the posterior part of the inner ankle bone. Massaging this
point can nourish the kidney yin, guide the kidney water, and
clear lung fire. Finally, I told him to hit the Zhongfu point
(which is the triangle depression outside the clavicle) with a
hollow fist to clear and harmonize lung energy.

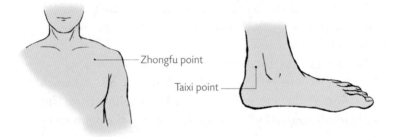

Zhongfu point

Taixi point

Rubbing the above areas and points relieves asthma and
cough and stops bleeding.

Doing these exercises 3–4 times a day and massaging each
point on both sides of the body 36 or 54 times would bring relief
to the elderly man's condition.

The three vital points and the thenar eminence are located
on both sides of the body. The whole exercise takes only seven to
eight minutes. If the patient can simultaneously practice the *xi*,
hu, *xu*, and *chui* breathing techniques (see pages 61, 63, 66 and
67) and take a happy walk (see page 90) for 40–50 minutes, the
effect of clearing lung heat can be achieved.

Asthma

Today, the incidence rate of bronchial asthma is increasing. Patients who suffer from bronchial asthma often have wheezing dyspnea, especially expiratory dyspnea, accompanied by agitation and a dull pain in the chest. By the time the condition has progressed to this state, most of the accessory respiratory muscles will have participated in the breathing movements, and there will be apparent depressions around the clavicles. In the most serious cases, the patient will open the mouth and raise the shoulders, sweating profusely all over, and their lips and fingers will turn purple. Some may also cough badly, coughing up a foamy phlegm.

Patients suffering from bronchial asthma look normal when they are not seized by the ailment. According to the vital energy transformation theory in traditional Chinese medicine, the lungs are the governor of energy and the kidneys are the root of energy. If poor kidney function is not improved, the energy the patient breathes in cannot be induced into the kidney, which will disturb the energy and block it inside the lung, resulting in asthma. Superficially, asthma is related to the lungs, but, in fact, it is connected to the kidneys. Thus, to cure asthma, we should focus on toning the kidneys and purging the lungs.

There is a tuck exercise effective in curing bronchial asthma. Before doing the exercise, the patient should use the *xi* breathing technique to exhale long and inhale short until he begins to sweat on the nose and upper lip. He should then take a happy walk to relax himself all over. After this, he is ready for the tuck exercise.

The exercise consists of first lying on the back on a bed, bending the knees and tucking the body inward with hands clasped around the shins. Lower the head, with the lower jaw tucked tightly against the chest, the thighs against the abdomen, and the waist touching the bed. After inhaling deeply, clasp your hands around your knees and hold your breath until it reaches your waist. When you can hold your breath no more, release your hands and stretch your legs. Straighten your waist and neck and use the *chui* breathing technique (see page 66) to exhale, then inhale and tuck your body inward.

Stand up with your feet together. Relax all over, squat with bended knees and with your hands clasped just below the knees. Keep your thighs tucked tightly against your chest and abdomen, bend your neck and lower your head to keep them as close to the knees as possible. Concentrate your mind on the Mingmen point.

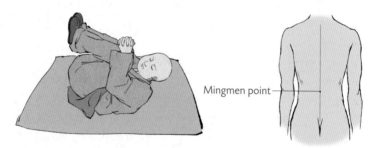

Mingmen point

When breathing, you must pay attention and inhale as you squat, then lower your head and hold your breath until it reaches the waist. When you can hold your breath no more, straighten your back and get on your feet, then exhale using the *chui* breathing technique. Repeat this at least six times.

Alternatively, stand with your feet together and your back bent forward. Pull your heels with your hands and take a deep breath, holding it until it reaches your waist. When you can hold your breath no more, straighten your back and exhale using the *chui* breathing technique.

This exercise is fit for both old and young. If you can persevere, your health will improve. Gradually, when the positive energy in your body can control the negative energy, your asthma will naturally be relieved.

Pulmonary Dust Contamination
Traffic police and teachers are exposed to car fumes and chalk

dust every day. They sacrifice their health for others' safety and growth. Once when I was working in the hospital, I encountered a middle school teacher whose X-ray test showed some reticulate shadows in the middle and lower lobes of his lung.

People who are often exposed to dust can do an exercise to prevent dust pollution and enhance their health. The exercise is very simple. Expand the chest while walking backwards. Walking backwards can mobilize the energy and blood throughout the body, and expanding the chest can help diffuse the inhibited lung energy and relieve stuffiness in the chest.

For safety's sake, we must do this exercise on a broad, and flat surface, because when we walk backwards, we cannot see what is behind us. To start, we can practice walking backwards, then when we are familiar with it, we can expand our chest while walking. In addition, those who suffer from high blood pressure and dizziness should not do this exercise.

I asked the teacher to practice this method. Three months later, he came back again to have an X-ray of his lungs, which showed that the reticulate shadows had disappeared. Of course, this exercise was effective for him in part because his symptoms were not serious. But even for patients with more serious conditions, it can inhibit the progression of the disease.

Chronic Pharyngitis

Ms. Huang, 36, was a well-known opera actress with a troupe in Henan Province. When she consulted with me, she said, "This is the peak of my career, but I have recently contracted chronic pharyngitis. My throat itches, and I can't clear it. This has seriously affected my work. It has caused me to miss several performances with the troupe."

"If you can follow the two thing I will teach you, you will surely recover," I said.

The first method was to buy 10 g of smoked plums and 50 g of olives, wash them clean, and put them into an earthenware pot. Add water into the pot until the ingredients are fully submerged. Soak the content in water for a whole day, then boil it over fire. Continue to boil it for a dozen minutes after the water starts boiling. Add sugar to taste and finish drinking it within one day.

This prescription clears the throat, disinhibits the diaphragm, relieves cough, and reduces sputum. In fact, most people's pharyngitis is not serious. They simply feel uncomfortable in the throat, as if there were some foreign substance there. This decoction can greatly refresh the throat.

The second method is to protect the throat. Be careful not to expose the throat to cold or chill. Wear a scarf when you go outdoors.

Ms. Huang followed these methods and recovered within seven days.

5. Other Diseases

Today, medical specializations have become more and more specified, and so have the doctors' field of expertise. This is very bad, because, for many diseases, their sites of pathological change are not in the same place as the symptoms, and their causes are diverse. For example, bile reflux makes the patient have a bitter feeling in the mouth, and a pain in the leg may be caused by the compression of the lumbar nerves.

In this sense, we say we do not advocate the method of treating the head when it aches and treating the foot when it hurts. To become an exceptional doctor, we should be able to keep an eye on the overall picture.

Nephritis

More than 20 years ago, Mr. Chen came to me to treat his high blood pressure. While making my diagnosis, I suddenly noticed that his eyelids were swollen. I immediately became alarmed and asked, "How long have your eyelids been swollen?"

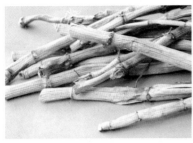

Cogongrass rhizome.

"Just today," answered Mr. Chen. "I noticed it this morning when I was combing my hair. I was wondering why it became like that, since I did not stay up late last night."

I immediately said, "You might have acute nephritis. For safety's sake, go and have a routine urianlysis."

Ten minutes later, Mr. Chen came back to my office. I was astonished, because the test result could not possibly have come out so quickly. Unexpectedly, in a bit of a panic, he told me that the test result was not out yet, but he found blood in his urine when he had gone to the toilet.

Another ten minutes passed before the test results came out, and they showed that there were white cells in his urine, an obvious sign of acute nephritis.

"Don't panic," I told him. "You'll be fine after taking some medicine that invigorates the kidneys and removes dampness." I wrote down a prescription.

Ingredients: Cogongrass rhizome (25 g, 100 g if it is fresh), fresh waxgourd peel (50 g), watermelon peel (50 g), red beans (50 g) and rice (150 g) .

Cooking method: Wrap the first three ingredients tightly in a gauze bag and boil it in water with red beans. Continue to boil it for about 20 minutes after the water starts to boil. Take out the bag, add rice to the water and boil it for another 20 minutes.

Eat the soup in the morning and evening.

Cogongrass rhizome cools the blood, stops bleeding, reduces fever, and causes diuresis. Waxgourd peel induces diuresis to alleviate edema. Watermelon peel promotes urination. Red beans are very effective in treating renal edema.

The entire prescription is focused on alleviating edema, promoting urination, and stopping bleeding.

After taking the medicine for a day, Mr. Chen's eyelids were no longer swollen. He continued to take it for three more days, then came to my office on the fourth day. I asked him to do a routine urianlysis again, which showed that his indexes had returned to normal.

Chronic Cholecystitis

According to the *Inner Canon of the Yellow Emperor*, the gallbladder can adjust balance. If you keep eating irregularly or are prone to anger, you may easily have cholecystitis or even gallstones.

Ms. Yang suffered from chronic cholecystitis. She often felt pain in her right upper quadrant, which grew more frequent after meals. Things seemed to have gotten worse recently. She felt sick every time she ate, and the pain often radiated all the way to her right scapula. In addition, the pain lasted longer and longer. What had lasted several minutes in the past now lasted several dozen minutes, or even more than an hour.

She went to a doctor two months earlier, but to no avail. I read her previous case report and test results. The ultrasonic B test showed that she had quicksand-like gallstones, which, fortunately, were not hard gallstones with super echoes. She had pain in the bladder because the flow of bile after meals made the gallstones move, which stimulated the gall bladder wall or bile duct.

In this case, apart from treating cholecystitis, we also needed to remove the stones to prevent them from becoming increasingly harder and larger, making it more difficult to remove them.

In Zen medicine, there is an effective method for removing gallstones, which I once taught to many patients with cholecystitis plus gallstones. The method includes first taking a happy walk (see page 90) ten minutes after each meal, then practicing at least six rounds of *hu* and *xu* breathing techniques (see pages 61 and 63). Since cholecystitis relates most closely to the liver and stomach, the *hu* breathing technique will promote the flow of energy and sooth the liver, and the *xu* breathing technique nourishes the spleen and stomach. After these are completed, find a place with fresh air and stand there to do two groups of movements.

The first group of movements: Stamp the heels, stand with your feet together, relax all over, and breathe naturally. Hold the fingers tightly together, stretch the fingertips forward, and place them on the upper part of your sides, with the arms reaching as far backwards as possible. Raise the heel as high as possible, then drop it abruptly.

The second group of movements: While stamping your feet, rub both sides of your body with your palms facing forward, thinking of your bladder as you move. Practice this movement 20–30 times daily.

After doing the exercise for a week, Ms. Yang's cholecystitis was greatly relieved. A month later, it had stopped breaking out altogether. Two months later, when she had her gallbladder reexamined, the quicksand-like gallstones had completely disappeared.

Cholecystitis and gallstones often go hand in hand. If treated in time, both can be cured. Otherwise, they will go from bad to worse, until finally the stones grow increasingly larger and harder. When the stones cannot be discharged from the bile duct, they must be removed surgically.

Pelvic Congestion Syndrome
After giving birth to her child, Ms. Yuan became sick. She told me at her consultation, "I haven't worked for six years, ever since my child was born." When I asked her about the cause of her disease, she told me the symptoms, pointing at her waist, abdomen, and hips. All her symptoms conformed to pelvic

congestion syndrome, a pain pressing downward in the pelvic cavity, a low-position backache, dyspareunia, menorrhagia, and leukorrhagia. I told her a very effective exercise to cure her disease. As long as she did it 6 times every day, she would fully recover. I record that exercise below.

❶ Lie on your back in the bed and bend your knees. Keeping your upper body motionless, twist your hip joint to the left, moving your knees as far left as possible, then inhale. Twist your hip joint and move your knees to the right, then exhale. Repeat this set of movements at least 40 times. Be careful to keep your scapula on the bed when you twist.

❷ Straighten your legs and relax your abdomen. Place your left hand horizontally below the xiphoid, rub to the right and downward toward the area above the pubic symphysis, then rub to the left and upward toward the area below the xiphoid. Exhale as you rub to the right and downward, and inhale when you rub to the left and upward. Repeat this set of movements 100 times. After that, use your right hand to rub in the same pattern another 100 times, but in opposite directions.

❸ Regulate your breathing and rest for a little while. Then bend your knees, tuck your body, lower your head, and hold your knees tightly with both hands, with your head touching your knees (don't worry if your head cannot touch your knees at first) and your waist on the bed. Inhale as you lie on your back and hold your breath as you tuck your body and hold your knees. Then relax your hands, straighten your legs, lower your head, and resume the lying posture. Repeat this set of movements at least 6 times.

❹ Contract your anus and vulva while inhaling and loose them while exhaling. This is similar to the levator ani movement. Repeat this set of movements at least 30 times.

Appendices

Illustrations of Meridians

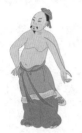
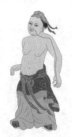
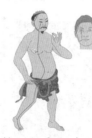
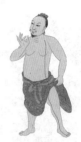

Taiyin Lung Meridian of Hand (LU)

Yangming Large Intestine Meridian of Hand (LI)

Yangming Stomach Meridian of Foot (ST)

Taiyin Spleen Meridian of Foot (SP)

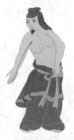
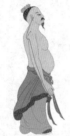
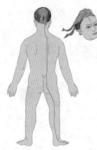
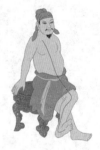

Shaoyin Heart Meridian of Hand (HT)

Taiyang Small Intestine Meridian of Hand (SI)

Taiyang Bladder Meridian of Foot (BL)

Shaoyin Kidney Meridian of Foot (KI)

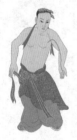
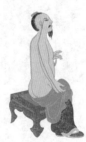
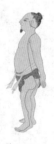
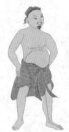
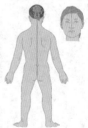

Jueyin Pericardium Meridian of Hand (PC)

Shaoyang Sanjiao Meridian of Hand (SJ)

Shaoyang Gallbladder Meridian of Foot (GB)

Jueyin Liver Meridian of Foot (LV)

Governing Vessel (DU)

According to traditional Chinese medicine, there are 12 meridian and collateral channels, together with the Conception and Governing vessels inside the human body. A total of 365 acupuncture points are arranged along them.

Index